Register Now for Online Access to Your Book!

Your print purchase of *Handbook of Prostate Cancer and Other Genitourinary Malignancies*, **includes online access to the contents of your book**—increasing accessibility, portability, and searchability!

Access today at:

http://connect.springerpub.com/content/book/978-1-6170-5286-6
or scan the QR code at the right with your smartphone
and enter the access code below.

CMYU6BN6

Scan here for quick access.

If you are experiencing problems accessing the digital component of this product, please contact our customer service department at cs@springerpub.com

The online access with your print purchase is available at the publisher's discretion and may be removed at any time without notice.

Publisher's Note: New and used products purchased from third-party sellers are not guaranteed for quality, authenticity, or access to any included digital components.

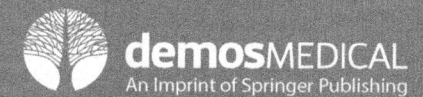

View all our products at springerpub.com/demosmedical

Handbook of Prostate Cancer and Other Genitourinary Malignancies

Editors

Teresa Gray Hayes, MD, PhD
Associate Professor of Medicine, Emeritus
Internal Medicine/Hematology-Oncology
Baylor College of Medicine
Houston, Texas

Martha Pritchett Mims, MD, PhD
Associate Professor and Chief of Hematology and Oncology
Internal Medicine/Hematology-Oncology
Baylor College of Medicine
Houston, Texas

Jennifer Marie Taylor, MD, MPH
Assistant Professor
Urology
Baylor College of Medicine;
Staff Surgeon, Urology
Michael E. DeBakey VA Medical Center
Houston, Texas

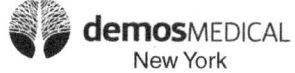

Visit our website at www.demosmedical.com

ISBN: 9781620701096
e-book ISBN: 9781617052866

Acquisitions Editor: David D'Addona
Compositor: diacriTech

Copyright © 2017 Springer Publishing Company.
Demos Medical Publishing is an imprint of Springer Publishing Company, LLC.

All rights reserved. This book is protected by copyright. No part of it may be reproduced, stored in a retrieval system, or transmitted in any form or by any means, electronic, mechanical, photocopying, recording, or otherwise, without the prior written permission of the publisher.

Medicine is an ever-changing science. Research and clinical experience are continually expanding our knowledge, in particular our understanding of proper treatment and drug therapy. The authors, editors, and publisher have made every effort to ensure that all information in this book is in accordance with the state of knowledge at the time of production of the book. Nevertheless, the authors, editors, and publisher are not responsible for errors or omissions or for any consequences from application of the information in this book and make no warranty, expressed or implied, with respect to the contents of the publication. Every reader should examine carefully the package inserts accompanying each drug and should carefully check whether the dosage schedules mentioned therein or the contraindications stated by the manufacturer differ from the statements made in this book. Such examination is particularly important with drugs that are either rarely used or have been newly released on the market.

Library of Congress Cataloging-in-Publication Data
Names: Hayes, Teresa Gray, editor. | Mims, Martha Pritchett, editor. | Taylor, Jennifer Marie, editor.
Title: Handbook of prostate cancer and other genitourinary malignancies / editors, Teresa Gray Hayes, Martha Pritchett Mims, Jennifer Marie Taylor.
Description: New York: Demos Medical, [2017] | Includes bibliographical references and index.
Identifiers: LCCN 2017013587 | ISBN 9781620701096 | ISBN 9781617052866
Subjects: | MESH: Prostatic Neoplasms | Urogenital Neoplasms
Classification: LCC RC280.P7 | NLM WJ 762 | DDC 616.99/463—dc23
LC record available at https://lccn.loc.gov/2017013587

Contact us to receive discount rates on bulk purchases.
We can also customize our books to meet your needs.
For more information please contact: sales@springerpub.com

Printed in the United States of America by McNaughton & Gunn.
16 17 18 19 20 / 5 4 3 2 1

To our patients, who have taught us so much; and to our trainees, who have worked so hard to ensure that our patients get the best care possible.

Contents

Contributors xi
Preface xv
Acknowledgments xvii

I. Prostate Cancer

EARLY STAGE PROSTATE CANCER

1. Prostate Cancer Screening 3
   Thiri Khin and Nicholas Mitsiades

2. Management of Early Stage Prostate Cancer 9
   Pranav Dadhich and Jennifer Marie Taylor

3. Early Stage Prostate Cancer: Biochemical Relapse 21
   Andrew Jackson and Teresa Gray Hayes

4. Intermittent Androgen Ablation in Biochemical Relapse of Early Stage Prostate Cancer 27
   Chitra Balasundaram and Teresa Gray Hayes

5. Treatment of Therapy Complications 33
   Pranav Dadhich and Jennifer Marie Taylor

6. Early Stage Prostate Cancer: Controversies in Management 37
   Jianbo Wang and Teresa Gray Hayes

7. Early Stage Prostate Cancer Survivorship Challenges 43
   Andrew Jackson and Teresa Gray Hayes

MANAGEMENT OF ADVANCED PROSTATE CANCER

8. Treatment of Metastatic Cancer: Hormonal Agents, Chemotherapy, Immune Modulation, and Radiopharmaceuticals 47
   Jesus H. Hermosillo-Rodriguez and Teresa Gray Hayes

9. Intermittent Androgen Ablation in Metastatic Prostate Cancer 59
   Abhishek Marballi and Teresa Gray Hayes

10. Bone Health and Use of Adjunctive Agents   65
    Jesus H. Hermosillo-Rodriguez and Nicholas Mitsiades

11. Advanced Stage Prostate Cancer: Controversies in Management   69
    Jesus H. Hermosillo-Rodriguez and Nicholas Mitsiades

12. Advanced Prostate Cancer Survivorship Challenges and Issues   73
    Jesus H. Hermosillo-Rodriguez and Nicholas Mitsiades

II. Other Genitourinary Malignancies
KIDNEY CANCER

13. Kidney Cancer: Histologic Subtypes and Genetic Syndromes   79
    Thiri Khin and Teresa Gray Hayes

14. Treatment of Early Stage Renal Cell Carcinoma: Surgical Approaches, Partial Nephrectomy, and Ablation   89
    Friedrich-Carl von Rundstedt, Wesley A. Mayer, and Richard E. Link

15. Renal Cell Carcinoma: Treatment of Advanced Kidney Cancer   97
    Kanza S. Abbas and Teresa Gray Hayes

16. Controversies in the Surgical Management of Renal Cell Carcinoma   103
    Thomas E. Stout and Samit D. Soni

17. Investigational Technologies in the Surgical Management of Renal Cell Carcinoma   113
    Thomas E. Stout and Samit D. Soni

18. Kidney Cancer Survivorship Challenges and Issues   117
    Elaine Chang and Wesley A. Mayer

UPPER TRACT UROTHELIAL CANCER

19. Overview of Upper Tract Urothelial Cancers   123
    Harish Madala, Carli Calderone, and Wesley A. Mayer

20. Management of Early Stage Upper Tract Urothelial Cancers   135
    Harish Madala, Carli Calderone, and Wesley A. Mayer

21. Treatment of Metastatic Upper Tract Urothelial Cancers   141
    Jose Pacheco, Saleha Sajid, and Teresa Gray Hayes

22. Controversies in the Management of Upper Tract Urothelial Cancer   147
    Jose Pacheco and Jennifer Marie Taylor

23. Upper Tract Urothelial Carcinoma Survivorship *153*
    Spencer Craven and Jennifer Marie Taylor

    BLADDER CANCER

24. Urothelial Cancer of the Bladder: Treatment of Early Stage Disease *157*
    Carli Calderone and Jennifer Marie Taylor

25. Management of Invasive Bladder Cancer: Surgery, Chemotherapy, and Radiation Therapy *177*
    Arun Rai, Thiri Khin, Teresa Gray Hayes, and Jennifer Marie Taylor

26. Treatment of Metastatic Bladder Cancer: Chemotherapy and Checkpoint Inhibitors *197*
    Jose Pacheco and Teresa Gray Hayes

27. Controversies in the Management of Bladder Cancer *203*
    Jose Pacheco and Teresa Gray Hayes

28. Bladder Cancer Surveillance and Survivorship *209*
    Bethany R. Desroches and Jennifer Marie Taylor

    TESTICULAR CANCER

29. Seminomas *215*
    Mehmet Akce and Teresa Gray Hayes

30. Nonseminomatous Germ Cell Tumors: Early Stage, Late Stage *225*
    Ryan Yates and Martha Pritchett Mims

31. Reproductive Considerations and Long-Term Complications of Therapy *235*
    Thiri Khin and Martha Pritchett Mims

32. Controversies in the Management of Testicular Cancer *243*
    Ghana Kang and Martha Pritchett Mims

    PENILE CANCER

33. Treatment of Early Stage Penile Cancer *251*
    Guilherme Godoy

34. Treatment of Metastatic Penile Cancer: Chemotherapy *267*
    Abhishek Marballi and Teresa Gray Hayes

35. Controversies in the Management of Penile Cancer *273*
    Guilherme Godoy

36. Penile Cancer Survivorship Challenges and Issues *279*
    Spencer Craven and Guilherme Godoy

Index 283

Contributors

Kanza S. Abbas, MD
Clinical Postdoctoral Fellow
Internal Medicine/
 Hematology-Oncology
Baylor College of Medicine,
 Houston, Texas
Now at Kelsey Seybold Clinic,
 Houston, Texas

Mehmet Akce, MD
Clinical Postdoctoral Fellow
Internal Medicine/
 Hematology-Oncology
Baylor College of Medicine,
 Houston, Texas

Chitra Balasundaram, MD
Clinical Postdoctoral Fellow
Internal Medicine/
 Hematology-Oncology
Baylor College of Medicine,
 Houston, Texas
Now at Mercy Clinic Cancer
 and Hematology,
 Springfield, Missouri

Carli Calderone, MD
Medical Resident
Urology
Emory University,
 Atlanta, Georgia

Elaine Chang, MD
Clinical Postdoctoral Fellow
Internal Medicine/
 Hematology-Oncology
Baylor College of Medicine,
 Houston, Texas

Spencer Craven, MD
Medical Resident
Urology
Baylor College of Medicine,
 Houston, Texas

Pranav Dadhich, MD
Medical Student
Urology
Baylor College of Medicine,
 Houston, Texas

Bethany R. Desroches, MD
Medical Resident
Urology
Baylor College of Medicine,
 Houston, Texas

Guilherme Godoy, MD
Assistant Professor
Urology
Baylor College of Medicine,
 Houston, Texas

Teresa Gray Hayes, MD, PhD
Associate Professor of Medicine, Emeritus
Internal Medicine/
 Hematology-Oncology
Baylor College of Medicine,
 Houston, Texas

Jesus H. Hermosillo-Rodriguez, MD
Clinical Postdoctoral Fellow
Internal Medicine/
 Hematology-Oncology
Baylor College of Medicine,
 Houston, Texas
Now at Colorado Permanente
 Medical Group,
 Denver, Colorado

Andrew Jackson, MD
Clinical Postdoctoral Fellow
Internal Medicine/
 Hematology-Oncology
Baylor College of Medicine,
 Houston, Texas

Ghana Kang, MD
Clinical Postdoctoral Fellow
Internal Medicine/
 Hematology-Oncology
Baylor College of Medicine,
 Houston, Texas
Now at Northern Virginia
 Hematology Associates,
 Woodbridge, Virginia

Thiri Khin, MD
Clinical Postdoctoral Fellow
Internal Medicine/
 Hematology-Oncology
Baylor College of Medicine,
 Houston, Texas

Richard E. Link, MD
Associate Professor
Urology
Baylor College of Medicine,
 Houston, Texas

Harish Madala, MD
Clinical Postdoctoral Fellow
Internal Medicine/
 Hematology-Oncology
Baylor College of Medicine,
 Houston, Texas

Abhishek Marballi, MD
Clinical Postdoctoral Fellow
Internal Medicine/
 Hematology-Oncology
Baylor College of Medicine,
 Houston, Texas
Now at Crystal Run
 Healthcare,
 Middletown, New York

Wesley A. Mayer, MD
Assistant Professor
Urology
Baylor College of Medicine,
 Houston, Texas

Martha Pritchett Mims, MD, PhD
Associate Professor and
 Chief of Hematology and
 Oncology
Internal Medicine/
 Hematology-Oncology
Baylor College of Medicine,
 Houston, Texas

Nicholas Mitsiades, MD
Assistant Professor
Internal Medicine/
 Hematology-Oncology
Baylor College of Medicine,
 Houston, Texas

Jose Pacheco, MD
Clinical Postdoctoral Fellow
Internal Medicine/
 Hematology-Oncology
Baylor College of Medicine,
 Houston, Texas

Arun Rai, MD
Medical Resident
Urology
Baylor College of Medicine,
  Houston, Texas

Saleha Sajid, MBBS
Assistant Professor
Internal Medicine/
  Hematology-Oncology
Baylor College of Medicine,
  Houston, Texas
Now at Genesis Medical Group,
  Woodlands, Texas

Samit D. Soni, MD
Assistant Professor
Urology
Baylor College of Medicine,
  Houston, Texas

Thomas E. Stout, MD
Medical Student
Urology
Baylor College of Medicine,
  Houston, Texas

Jennifer Marie Taylor, MD, MPH
Assistant Professor
Urology
Baylor College of Medicine;
Staff Surgeon
Michael E. DeBakey VA Medical
  Center,
  Houston, Texas

Friedrich-Carl von Rundstedt, MD
Staff Physician
Urology
Jena University Hospital, Jena,
  Thuringia, Germany

Jianbo Wang, MB, PhD
Clinical Postdoctoral Fellow
Internal Medicine-
  Hematology-Oncology
Baylor College of Medicine,
  Houston, Texas

Ryan Yates, MD
Clinical Postdoctoral Fellow
Internal Medicine/
  Hematology-Oncology
Baylor College of Medicine,
  Houston, Texas

Preface

Genitourinary malignancies represent a wide spectrum of risk and prognosis. The last decade or more has brought an extraordinary evolution in outcomes for patients with these diseases at advanced stages, mainly through development and adoption of new systemic therapies. In addition, greater attention is being paid to comprehensive assessment of the patient before, during, and after treatment. More systematic measurement of influential medical and psychosocial factors has allowed for better treatment selection and symptom management.

This handbook aims to provide a broad overview and current summary of the state of assessment, diagnosis, and treatment of these malignancies. It will be useful for clinicians at multiple stages in medical and surgical specialties: in training, early in a career, and looking for updated information. With the ability to reference quickly for a specific question, or review a larger section all at once, the reader can customize the depth with which he or she uses the handbook.

This remains an exciting time for those dealing with many of these malignancies, with advances and innovations continuing in both the medical and surgical arenas. The dissemination of these developments and collaboration among specialists will continue to bring improved outcomes to our patients living with or surviving these diseases. We are grateful to the patients and providers who work together in clinical trials, which are the foundation of the progress and drive the evolution of the field forward.

We welcome your feedback and suggestions as you use this handbook in practice.

Jennifer Marie Taylor, MD, MPH

Acknowledgments

The authors would like to acknowledge Baylor College of Medicine and the Michael E. DeBakey VA Medical Center, Houston, Texas, for their support and assistance.

Prostate Cancer

EARLY STAGE PROSTATE CANCER

Prostate Cancer Screening

Thiri Khin and Nicholas Mitsiades

INTRODUCTION

Prostate cancer is the most common visceral cancer in the United States and the second leading cause of cancer death after lung cancer. In the United States, approximately one in seven men will be diagnosed with prostate cancer. One in 39 prostate cancer patients will die from the disease. Survival of prostate cancer is related to many factors, including age and stage at diagnosis (1). Although the 5-year survival rate for early localized prostate cancer is 100%, survival is only 29.3% for distant metastatic disease.

With the goal of reducing cancer-related morbidity and mortality by early detection, screening strategies are employed in common and lethal cancers such as prostate cancer. Prostate-specific antigen (PSA) was initially developed as a tumor marker to assess the extent of disease and detect treatment response. Despite a lack of efficacy data from randomized controlled trials (RCTs), PSA was incorporated into prostate cancer screening in the early 1990s, which subsequently lead to a peak increase in the detected incidence of prostate cancer. Most of the cancers detected were early stage disease, which otherwise would have not been discovered and may not have been clinically relevant. However, early detection often led to aggressive treatment. Since then, the benefits of PSA screening have been questioned and have been a major topic of debate among clinicians and guideline organizations.

VARIATIONS OF PSA LEVEL

PSA is a glycoprotein expressed in both normal and neoplastic prostatic epithelial tissue. The PSA level reflects the amount of prostate glandular epithelium in normal healthy men. Prostate size increases with age and in turn increases the PSA level. The PSA increases by 3.2% (0.04 ng/mL) per year for a 60-year old, and reference ranges for different age groups have been proposed.

In addition, multiple factors may influence the PSA level in healthy individuals. African American men have higher PSA levels when compared to White men. Prostatitis, perineal trauma, benign prostatic hypertrophy, prostate biopsy, and ejaculation can elevate the PSA level. Medications such as 5-alpha reductase inhibitors can reduce the PSA level by up to 50%. Nonsteroidal anti-inflammatory drugs (NSAIDs), acetaminophen, statins, and thiazide diuretics can lower the PSA level to varying degrees. Despite these variations, a traditional cutoff of 4 ng/mL or more has been considered abnormal by most clinicians.

PSA TESTING IN MALIGNANCY

PSA levels are raised in malignancy, not only due to increased production by malignant epithelial cells but also due to disruption of vasculature and release of PSA into the bloodstream. Multiple studies have shown that a rise in PSA precedes the development of prostate cancer by 5 to 10 years. Different cancers have varying levels of PSA elevation, and poorly differentiated cancer can have a large tumor burden with minimally elevated PSA.

Using a cutoff value of 4 ng/mL, the estimated sensitivity is 21% for detecting any prostate cancer and 51% for high-grade cancer in pooled analyses. Specificity is estimated to be 91%. Positive predictive value (PPV) is 30%, which means that one in three men with PSA more than 4 ng/mL has prostate cancer. Negative predictive value (NPV) is 85% for a PSA level lower than 4 ng/mL (2). Different strategies have been tested to improve the performance of PSA testing in prostate cancer. Lowering the cutoff level increases the sensitivity level but in turn reduces specificity. Various tests such as PSA velocity, PSA density, the ratio of free to total PSA, 4 Kallikrein tests (4Ktest), and [−2] ProPSA have been explored, and none of the tests have shown improvement in clinical outcomes.

DIGITAL RECTAL EXAMINATION

Digital rectal examination (DRE) is one of the oldest methods used to diagnose prostate cancer. DRE can detect tumors in the posterior and lateral aspects of the prostate gland. Because only 85% of prostate cancer is peripherally located, some cancers may be missed by DRE. A meta-analysis shows the positive predictive value of DRE is 28% with sensitivity 59% and specificity 95% (3). However, DRE is not recommended as a stand-alone method for screening of prostate cancer, since it is operator dependent and studies have shown no improvement in outcome with DRE screening alone. When combined with PSA testing, DRE can increase the rate of detection of prostate cancer by 1%, but combined PSA and DRE has not shown a benefit in reducing cancer morbidity and mortality.

IMPACT OF PROSTATE CANCER SCREENING

The efficacy of PSA screening has been investigated in multiple observational studies and RCTs. Two large RCTs, the European Randomized Study of Screening for Prostate Cancer (ERSPC) and the Prostate, Lung, Colorectal, and Ovarian (PLCO) screening trial performed in the United States, produced different outcomes and increased the controversy about prostate cancer screening.

The ERSPC trial, which spanned across seven centers in Europe, enrolled 182,160 men between the ages of 50 and 74 who were randomly assigned to PSA screening (an average of once every 4 years) or a control group without screening. With a follow-up of 13 years, prostate cancer mortality was reported to be 21% lower in the screening group than in the control group. The absolute risk reduction was 0.11 per 1,000 patient years between the two groups (4).

In the PLCO screening trial, 76,693 men between the ages of 55 and 74 were randomly assigned to annual screening with PSA and DRE or to usual care. In contrast to the ERSPC, there was no reduction in the primary outcome of prostate cancer mortality after 7 years of follow-up, and the 13-year update similarly showed no difference in mortality between the screening and control groups (5).

There were differences in the design of the two trials. The ERSPC trial was a combination of results from multiple centers across Europe. Different centers used DRE and transrectal ultrasonography and employed varying PSA cutoffs between 2.5 and 4 ng/mL. The majority of the centers used 3 ng/mL. In the PLCO trial, PSA was combined with DRE and the cutoff was set at 4 ng/mL. The overall rate of contamination PSA screening in the control group is not reported in the ERSPC trial. Up to 24% of patients with prostate cancer in the control arm did not undergo aggressive treatment with surgery or radiation in the ESRPC trial. The difference in treatment in both arms may explain the positive outcome in reducing cancer-related mortality. In the PLCO trial, the control group had a high contamination rate, with up to 80% of subjects receiving PSA screening, which might contribute to the null result.

RISKS ASSOCIATED WITH PROSTATE CANCER SCREENING

In both the ERSPC and PLCO trials, the incidence of cancer was higher in the screening group than in the control group. In the ERSPC trial, 24% of all cancers diagnosed were stage T1c, that is, clinically unapparent tumor detected by needle biopsy due to elevated PSA level. This highlights the possible overdiagnosis resulting from screening methods. Studies have shown that screening with PSA can lead to an overdiagnosis rate of up to 50%.

Many patients with early prostate cancer do not develop symptoms for many years. Some cancers are indolent, and many may not ever need treatment. However, diagnostic intervention and treatment-related complications are immediate, can be morbid, and can lead to both physical and psychological harm. An elevated PSA often leads to prostate biopsy, which can lead to complications such as infection and bleeding requiring hospitalization. Radical prostatectomy can cause urinary incontinence, sexual problems, and bowel dysfunction, and has an operative mortality from 0.1% to 1%. Radiation therapy can also cause erectile dysfunction up to 45%, urinary incontinence up to 16%, and bowel problems up to 25%.

PROSTATE CANCER SCREENING: DO OR DO NOT?

Currently, the United States Preventive Services Task Force (USPSTF) recommends against screening for prostate cancer. Given the contrasting reports and limitations of both ERSPC and PLCO trials, the benefit of prostate cancer screening is uncertain. Though cancer screening may benefit some patients by early detection and treatment, the number needed to treat is very high (781 in the ERSPC trial) to save one patient from prostate cancer–related death. Since the hazards of diagnostic tests and treatment potentially outweigh the benefits, it is very important to inform patients, and the decision to screen should not be taken lightly. The American Cancer Society (ACS) and American Urological Association (AUA) have both emphasized informed decision making and recommend against screening in patients with life expectancy less than 10 years (6).

In patients who have decided to get screened, ACS recommends screening with PSA and/or DRE beginning at the age of 50 and screening discussions at age 40 to 45 for high-risk patients such as African American men and men with a family history of a first degree relative with prostate cancer diagnosed earlier than age 65 (6). Referral for biopsy is indicated at a level above 4 ng/mL, although many experts suggest repeating levels several weeks later if the PSA is below 7 ng/mL.

Further studies are needed to develop new screening methods and identify potential groups of patients who would potentially benefit from screening with minimal risk.

KEY POINTS

- Prostate cancer screening is highly controversial.
- Screening should be individualized based on patient interest and degree of risk for developing prostate cancer.
- Screening is not recommended for men with life expectancy less than 10 years.

REFERENCES

1. Siegel RL, Miller KD, Jemal A. Cancer statistics, 2016. *CA Cancer J Clin.* 2016;66:7-30.
2. Gann PH, Hennekens CH, Stampfer MJ. A prospective evaluation of plasma prostate-specific antigen for detection of prostatic cancer. *JAMA.* 1995;273(4):289-294.
3. Hoogendam A, et al . The diagnostic value of digital rectal examination in primary care screening for prostate cancer: a meta-analysis. *Fam Pract.* 1999 Dec;16(6):621-626.
4. Schröder FH, Hugosson J, Roobol MJ, et al. Screening and prostate-cancer mortality in a randomized European study. *N Engl J Med.* 2009;360(13):1320-1328.
5. Andriole GL, Crawford ED, Grubb RL, et al. Mortality results from a randomized prostate-cancer screening trial. *N Engl J Med.* 2009;360(13):1310-1319.
6. Wolf AM, Wender RC, Etzioni RB, et al. American Cancer Society guideline for the early detection of prostate cancer: update 2010. *CA Cancer J Clin.* 2010;60(2):70-98.

Management of Early Stage Prostate Cancer

Pranav Dadhich and Jennifer Marie Taylor

INTRODUCTION

The landscape for prostate cancer management has seen a fundamental shift in the past two to three decades. Prior to the discovery of the biomarker prostate-specific antigen (PSA), indolent carcinomas were often asymptomatic and overlooked, and prostate cancer was only discovered at later stages. Since 1992, after PSA was employed as a gold standard screening tool, there was a stage migration whereby many prostate carcinomas are now detected at much earlier stages (1). There was a dramatic increase in definitive management of organ-confined disease by surgery or radiation following the advent of PSA screening, and the natural history of treated prostate cancer extended significantly. The change in the demographics of patients at diagnosis has resulted in new conversations about the management of early disease and continued surveillance. To date, the primary treatment options for early stage prostate cancer are active surveillance, radical prostatectomy, and radiation-based therapies.

Staging of prostate cancer follows the standard tumor, node, and metastasis (TNM) staging system (see Table 2.1) that provides an assessment of primary tumor pathology as well as metastasis of the disease. TNM "tumor" category is the clinical stage based on the physical exam findings by digital rectal examination (DRE). Three factors—Gleason score, clinical stage (American Joint Committee on Cancer [AJCC] T category), and PSA—have been established as strong predictors of clinical outcomes and are currently used for risk stratification, ranging from very-low-risk to high-risk classifications. The following two tables describe, in a more detailed manner, the staging of prostate cancer and risk classifications currently used (Tables 2.1a and b).

Multiple models and nomograms are utilized to estimate risk, including the Partin tables, D'Amico classification, National Comprehensive Cancer Network (NCCN) risk groupings, University of California at San Francisco-Cancer of the Prostate Risk Assessment (UCSF-CAPRA) scoring, and others. See Table 2.2 for commonly used risk groupings from NCCN.

Currently, the American Urological Association (AUA) guidelines for management of clinically localized prostate cancer (3) recommend radiographic staging for patients with a Gleason score greater than 7 or those with a PSA greater than 20 ng/mL. Studies include a CT of the abdomen and pelvis with contrast and bone scan. Given the extremely low chance of finding metastatic disease in patients with low-risk or very-low-risk disease, radiographic staging studies are not recommended in those patients.

PET scan with fluorodeoxyglucose (FDG) has no role in initial staging of prostate cancer, as prostate malignancy has a highly variable avidity for FDG. If a patient with metastatic disease has FDG avidity in the primary prostate gland, a PET scan can help elucidate metastatic disease; however, it is not generally used in prostate adenocarcinoma. There are multiple newer molecular tests available for additional risk stratification and these may prove to be very useful in the prognostic counseling of patients either before or after definitive treatment. Each has a slightly different role, whether after biopsy, or after prostatectomy. Tests such as Myriad Prolaris, Decipher, and OncotypeDX may better individualize the discussion of risk and prognosis with a given patient. Studies are ongoing to examine the benefits and cost considerations of these tests.

ACTIVE SURVEILLANCE

The diagnosis of prostate cancer at earlier stages led to the consideration that many cancers being diagnosed may be indolent or low risk, without a need for immediate definitive treatment. Currently the average age at diagnosis is 66 years old. Modern cancer statistics confirm that 5-year relative survival is greater than 99% in men diagnosed with localized prostate cancer (4). This stage migration led to the development of active surveillance (AS) protocols for specific

Table 2.1 (a) AJCC Staging of Prostate Cancer, AJCC 8th Edition, 2017

AJCC Prostate Cancer Stage Groupings

	I		IIA		IIB	IIC	IIIA	IIIB	IIIC	IVA	IVB
Jewett-Whitmore stage	A1		A2, B0-2				C1-3			D1	D2
TNM stage	cT1a-c, cT2a N0M0	pT2 N0M0	cT1a-c, cT2a N0M0	cT2b-c N0M0	T1-2 N0M0	T1-2 N0M0	T1-2 N0M0	T3-4 N0M0	Any T N0M0	Any T N1M0	Any T N0M1
Grade group*	1	1	1	1	2	3, 4	1–4	1–4	5	Any	Any
PSA level (ng/mL)	<10	<10	≥10 <20	<20	<20	<20	≥20	Any	Any	Any	Any

AJCC, American Joint Committee on Cancer; PSA, prostate-specific antigen; TNM, tumor, node, and metastasis.

Source: Modified from Ref. (2). NCCN Clinical Practice Guidelines in Oncology (NCCN Guidelines). Prostate cancer, version 3, 2016. https://www.nccn.org/professionals/physician_gls/pdf/prostate.pdf. Accessed November 10, 2016.

* Grade Group is based on Gleason score and the two most common histologic patterns in the tissue specimen (see Table 2.1 (b))

Table 2.1 (b) Grade Group, which is Based on Gleason Score and Histologic Patterns

Grade Group	Gleason Score (Primary and Secondary Patterns)
1	≤6 (≤3 + 3)
2	7 (3 + 4)
3	7 (4 + 3)
4	8 (4 + 4)
5	9 or 10 (4 + 5, 5 + 4, or 5 + 5)

Table 2.2 NCCN Risk Stratification of Prostate Cancer Pretreatment

Risk profile	Criteria
Very low risk	• Clinical stage T1c • Gleason score ≤6 • PSA <10 ng/mL • Fewer than three biopsy cores positive, ≤50% cancer in any core • PSA density <0.15 ng/mL/g
Low risk	• Clinical stage T1a or T2a • Gleason score ≤6 • PSA <10 ng/mL
Intermediate risk (Any of three)	• Clinical stage T2b–T2c • Gleason score 7 • PSA 10–20 ng/mL
High risk (Any of three)	• Clinical stage T3a • Gleason score 8–10 • PSA >20 ng/mL
Very high risk	• Clinical stage T3b–T4 • Primary Gleason pattern 5 • >4 cores with Gleason score 8–10

NCCN, National Comprehensive Cancer Network; PSA, prostate-specific antigen.

Source: Adapted from Refs. (2, 3).

prostate cancer patients. The observation of earlier diagnosis of many cases of prostate cancer, leading to increasing rates of definitive treatment, raised the question of overtreatment, with an increased burden on the health care system and, more importantly, unnecessary side effects on a man's quality of life. When the predicted risk of progression, metastasis, or death from prostate cancer is outweighed by the risks of treatment-related morbidity, AS offers an alternative with proper patient education and counseling. Patients are eligible for AS based on features of stage, grade, and PSA and monitored with semiannual PSA coupled with DRE and repeat prostate biopsy or biopsies (5). Men with very-low-risk and low-risk disease can be candidates for AS, but most men with intermediate and all men with high-risk disease should be offered definitive treatment. Currently, our institution specifies number of positive biopsy cores, percentage of any positive core, Gleason score, PSA, and clinical stage as eligibility criteria, and we mandate an "enrollment" biopsy within 6 months and an MRI when possible to rule out missed higher-risk disease. Recent studies show that elderly patients with multiple comorbidities and low-risk to even intermediate-risk disease generally do not benefit from immediate definitive intervention (6). Criteria for enrollment continue to evolve, and in some cases and centers may be age stratified. The integration of MRI data, as well as newer molecular tests, may further refine the selection and participation of patients in AS protocols.

Data from institutional registries of patients on AS continue to mature, reinforcing the safety and viability of this management. Recent data from a prospective AS cohort in Toronto reported that among 993 patients on AS, 2.8% developed metastatic disease, including 15 men (1.5% of all patients) who died of prostate cancer after a median follow-up time of 9.6 years. Furthermore, there is good retention of patients on AS, with 27% having elected intervention in the follow-up period (median 6.4 years, range 0.2–19 years) (7). AS continues to gain traction as data provide compelling results that this treatment modality, when used correctly, can have excellent clinical outcomes (8).

AS may not be the best choice for patients likely to have a higher-risk disease due to genetic predisposition or family history. Clinicians must also be wary regarding differences in patient demographics, which could bias the results of studies and decrease their relevance to local populations.

The main fear for both providers and patients lies in the imperfect ability to define aggressive disease and predict future outcomes without a surgical specimen. Clinicians must work closely with patients to counsel them properly and agree on a decision with shared responsibility. A multitude of unique factors can affect the rate and degree of disease progression, and patients also have varying personal thresholds for intervention; thus, AS provides a good model for shared decision-making and prospective analysis of patient-reported outcomes.

RADICAL PROSTATECTOMY

Radical prostatectomy has evolved as the standard of care for definitive treatment in properly selected men with prostate cancer and adequate life expectancy. More advanced open surgical techniques and increased utilization of minimally invasive approaches have allowed for improved oncologic efficacy and reduction in complications and side effects.

Both data and marketing have driven the adoption of minimally invasive prostate surgery in the United States, where the vast majority of prostate cancer surgeries are now being performed via the robotic-assisted laparoscopic approach. Data show that robotic-assisted laparoscopic prostatectomy cases are associated with lower volume of blood loss, lower rate of blood transfusion, shorter length of hospital stay, and reduced use of postoperative narcotic analgesia (9). However, most studies stress that the oncologic and functional outcomes are more surgeon dependent than technique dependent. Cost-effectiveness studies suggest savings in high-volume centers, but the startup and maintenance costs are significant with a robotic system (10). Thus, open surgery continues to be a viable option in areas that lack access to robotics and remains the technique of choice in certain cases with increased complexity or risk.

Removal of the prostate allows physicians to eliminate the primary organ of disease and yields more prognostic information with pathologic analysis of the specimen. A regional (bilateral pelvic) lymph node dissection is performed in almost all cases to gain additional diagnostic and prognostic accuracy (11). It also may have a therapeutic benefit, even in cases of node positivity (12). Technical questions remain regarding the extent or anatomic limits of the dissection, and mapping studies have helped establish the most common expected routes of lymphatic dissemination (13). A bilateral node dissection is required in all cases, due to the crossing vascular and lymphatic drainage. Often, surgeons choose between a "standard" or "extended" template for dissection, depending on the presurgical risk of lymph node involvement, which can be predicted by surgical nomograms using clinical characteristics.

Open and robotic prostatectomy are generally associated with short (1–2 day) hospital stays and relatively rapid return to baseline functional status. A recent meta-analysis of 110 papers reporting robotic prostatectomy outcomes reported a mean rate of any complication of 9% (14). The most prevalent complications were lymphocele (3.1%), urine leak (1.8%), and reoperation (1.6%), and perioperative mortality rates between 0.02% and 0.5%. The incidence of major (Clavien 3–5) complications is quite low after prostatectomy, but patients most often notice and deal with the more lingering side effects of incontinence and erectile dysfunction. Return of continence and erectile function may take months to several years depending on preoperative function and recovery.

After modern radical prostatectomy, the rates of recurrence and metastasis vary dramatically by stage. Cancers with high pathologic Gleason scores (sum 8–10) are likely to recur, with up to 80% of men with biochemical recurrence. However, cancer-specific survival is excellent, up to 90% at 15 years, when the disease is organ-confined at time of resection (15). Prostate cancer-specific mortality after prostatectomy at 15 years ranges from 0.8% to 1.5% with organ-confined disease to 22% to 30% with node-positive disease (16). The indications for surgical management continue to expand to include higher-risk disease, with proper discussion of the likely need for multimodal treatment over the course of a man's illness.

RADIATION THERAPY

Radiation therapy (RT) to the prostate can be delivered through multiple modalities, including external beam RT (EBRT) and brachytherapy. EBRT has long been used as a means of combating genitourinary (GU) malignancy but has improved in terms of accuracy and precision secondary to technological advancements. Most recently, Intensity

Modulated Radiation Therapy (IMRT) as a form of EBRT has emerged as the treatment modality of choice. IMRT provides an exceptional capability to minimize the degree of scatter radiation to surrounding GU structures. The most relevant factors for determining eligibility for RT include PSA, Gleason score, and AJCC clinical stage. In addition, comorbidities, performance status, and urinary and sexual symptoms must be factored into the decision.

Conventional RT may be used even for higher-risk or non-organ confined disease, but data strongly support administration of androgen deprivation therapy (ADT) with RT for varying lengths of time in men with cancers having higher risk features (17,18). RT can also be given in lower doses to the pelvic node distribution or beyond the confines of the prostate capsule in carefully selected higher risk patients. Alongside the adoption of EBRT, brachytherapy has also seen its role continue to be relevant. Brachytherapy is generally used in men at lower stages and risk categories, as compared to EBRT, but some centers integrate EBRT and brachytherapy for higher risk cases. Two of the key focuses of brachytherapy involve ensuring proper implant placement and calculating the proper dose to be given over the proper interval of time.

Short-term side effects of radiation include urinary tract inflammation, gastrointestinal (GI) dysfunction, and erectile dysfunction, but the patient avoids some of the major morbidity risks associated with surgery. The more common long-term side effects include urinary dysfunction, reduced bladder compliance and capacity, urethral stricture, GI dysfunction (proctitis, urgency), hemorrhagic cystitis, and increased risk for secondary malignancy (19).

Cancer-specific recurrence and survival rates following RT continue to be studied. With refinements in technique, we continue to see improved oncologic efficacy and reduced side effects. The continued evolution of techniques has made direct survival comparisons of surgery to RT difficult due to the long natural history of treated prostate cancer, but for men with shorter life expectancies, significant comorbidity burdens, or personal concerns regarding risks, RT remains a mainstay alternative to surgery.

Posttreatment surveillance is most often done using a combination of prostate biopsy and PSA, the latter of which has been shown to be the most reliable predictor of local or distant relapse. In order to strive for even greater reductions in scatter radiation and subsequent side effects, clinicians have begun to study the use of focal radiotherapy, such as stereotactic body radiation therapy, or CyberKnife. Although focal radiation may spare tissues the burden of whole-gland radiation, there is some risk given the multifocal nature of prostate cancer.

FOCAL ABLATION AND MULTIMODAL USE OF RADIATION

There are additional modalities, including whole gland cryotherapy, whole gland high-intensity focused ultrasound (HIFU), and other less common techniques that aim to destroy malignant cells with maximal preservation of adjacent healthy tissues. Cryotherapy is available as primary therapy for low-risk to intermediate-risk organ-confined disease and is an established mode of salvage therapy for organ-confined biopsy-proven recurrence after radiation. Prostate ablation with HIFU has recently been Food and Drug Administration (FDA) approved and is being actively studied in the primary and salvage treatment spaces.

RT can also be offered following radical prostatectomy as either adjuvant or salvage radiation. Adjuvant radiation is utilized in the patient with high-risk pathologic features with an undetectable PSA nadir, whereas salvage radiation is offered to a patient with persistently detectable PSA or with biochemical recurrence after prostatectomy. National guidelines jointly written by the AUA and American Society of Radiation Oncology detail the decision process for selecting adjuvant or salvage RT after prostatectomy (20). The decision is a balance of risk of side effects of additional unnecessary therapy weighed against the risk of cancer progression.

Surgical intervention after primary RT becomes a much more complex surgery due to risks associated with salvage surgery on irradiated tissues, but in centers with experience, this remains a viable option for controlling localized recurrence after RT.

Table 2.3 Summary of Main Treatment Modalities for Localized Disease

Treatment modality	Patient selection	Major risks	Options after primary treatment failure
Active surveillance	• Very-low-risk or low-risk disease • Compliance with surveillance protocol	• Progression of organ-confined disease • Development of metastasis	• Any definitive therapy
Radical prostatectomy	• Resectable disease • Life expectance >10 y • Lower burden of comorbidity	• Urinary incontinence • Erectile dysfunction • Risks of major surgical procedure	• Adjuvant or salvage RT • ADT
RT	• Organ-confined disease • Multiple medical comorbidities • Poor surgical candidacy	• Irritative bowel or bladder dysfunction • Radiation cystitis • Urethral stricture • Erectile dysfunction	• Salvage surgery (highly selected candidates) • Salvage ablation • ADT
Whole gland ablation	• Low- to intermediate-risk disease • Organ-confined disease • Salvage treatment after failure of RT	• Similar to risks associated with RT but with lower probabilities of occurrence	• Salvage RT • ADT
Focal ablation	• Low-risk disease • Should only be in setting of clinical trial	• Treatment failure • Local side effects	• Definitive whole gland treatment: surgery, RT, whole gland ablation

ADT, androgen deprivation therapy; RT, radiation therapy.

> **KEY POINTS**
>
> - As the early management of prostate cancer continues to advance, clinicians must remain aware of the changing landscape of the treatment modalities available to their patients.
> - Mainstays for management of organ-confined disease are active surveillance, radical prostatectomy, and radiation therapy.
> - Focal ablation therapies remain an active area of investigation in the setting of clinical trials.

REFERENCES

1. Lu-Yao GL, Greenberg ER. Changes in prostate cancer incidence and treatment in USA. *Lancet.* 1994;343(8892):251-254.
2. NCCN Clinical Practice Guidelines in Oncology (NCCN Guidelines). Prostate cancer, version 2.2017. https://www.nccn.org/professionals/physician_gls/pdf/prostate.pdf. Accessed April 7, 2017.
3. Thompson I, Thrasher JB, Aus G, et al. Guideline for the management of clinically localized prostate cancer: 2007 update. *J Urol.* 2007;177(6):2106-2131.
4. Siegel RL, Miller KD, Jemal A. Cancer statistics, 2016. *CA Cancer J Clin.* 2016;66(1):7-30.
5. Tosoian JJ, Carter HB, Lepor A, Loeb S. Active surveillance for prostate cancer: current evidence and contemporary state of practice. *Nat Rev Urol.* 2016;13(4):205-215.
6. Stangelberger A, Waldert M, Djavan B. Prostate cancer in elderly men. *Rev Urol.* 2008;10(2):111-119.
7. Klotz L, Vesprini D, Sethukavalan P, et al. Long-term follow-up of a large active surveillance cohort of patients with prostate cancer. *J Clin Oncol.* 2015;33(3):272-277.
8. Cooperberg MR, Carroll PR. Trends in management for patients with localized prostate cancer, 1990–2013. *JAMA.* 2015;314(1):80-82.
9. Finkelstein J, Eckersberger E, Sadri H, et al. Open versus laparoscopic versus robot-assisted laparoscopic prostatectomy: the European and US experience. *Rev Urol.* 2010;12(1):35-43.

10. Barzi A, Klein EA, Dorff TB, et al. Prostatectomy at high-volume centers improves outcomes and lowers the costs of care for prostate cancer. *Prostate Cancer Prostatic Dis.* 2016;19(1):84-91.
11. Siemens DR. Why all prostate cancer surgery should include an adequate lymph node dissection. *Can Urol Assoc J.* 2010;4(6):427-429.
12. Touijer KA, Mazzola CR, Sjoberg DD, et al. Long-term outcomes of patients with lymph node metastasis treated with radical prostatectomy without adjuvant androgen-deprivation therapy. *Eur Urol.* 2014;65(1):20-25.
13. Nguyen DP, Huber PM, Metzger TA, et al. A specific mapping study using fluorescence sentinel lymph node detection in patients with intermediate- and high-risk prostate cancer undergoing extended pelvic lymph node dissection. *Eur Urol.* 2016;70(5):734-737.
14. Novara G, Ficarra V, Rosen RC, et al. Systematic review and meta-analysis of perioperative outcomes and complications after robot-assisted radical prostatectomy. *Eur Urol.* 2012;62(3):431-452.
15. Pierorazio PM, Guzzo TJ, Han M, et al. Long-term survival after radical prostatectomy for men with high Gleason sum in pathologic specimen. *Urology.* 2010;76(3):715-721.
16. Eggener SE, Scardino PT, Walsh PC, et al. Predicting 15-year prostate cancer specific mortality after radical prostatectomy. *J Urol.* 2011;185(3):869-875.
17. Lei J-H, Liu L-R, Wei Q, et al. Androgen-deprivation therapy alone versus combined with radiation therapy or chemotherapy for non-localized prostate cancer: a systematic review and meta-analysis. *Asian J Androl.* 2016;18(1):102-107.
18. Martin NE, D'Amico AV. Progress and controversies: radiation therapy for prostate cancer. *CA Cancer J Clin.* 2014;64(6):389-407.
19. Michaelson MD, Cotter SE, Gargollo PC, et al. Management of complications of prostate cancer treatment. *CA Cancer J Clin.* 2008;58(4):196-213.
20. Valicenti RK, Thompson I, Albertsen P, et al. Adjuvant and salvage radiation therapy after prostatectomy: American Society for Radiation Oncology/American Urological Association guidelines. *Int J Radiat Oncol Biol Phys.* 2013;86(5):822-828.

Early Stage Prostate Cancer: Biochemical Relapse 3

Andrew Jackson and Teresa Gray Hayes

INTRODUCTION

After definitive treatment of localized prostate cancer, routine monitoring of serum prostate-specific antigen (PSA) for early detection of relapse of disease is common practice. This frequently results in finding a rising PSA in the absence of detectable local or distant disease, which is termed biochemical relapse. Evaluation and subsequent management of rising PSA after treatment of localized prostate cancer is dependent on the original treatment modality.

BIOCHEMICAL RELAPSE AFTER RADICAL PROSTATECTOMY

After radical prostatectomy, all prostate tissues should have been removed and therefore PSA should not be detectable in the serum postoperatively. The American Urological Association (AUA) defines biochemical recurrence as serum PSA of greater than 0.2 ng/mL after prostatectomy in the absence of systemic disease (1). In cases where the postprostatectomy serum PSA does not decrease to undetectable levels or cases of early biochemical relapse with rapid PSA rise, one should suspect systemic disease rather than biochemical-only recurrence.

BIOCHEMICAL RELAPSE AFTER RADIATION THERAPY

Defining biochemical recurrence after radiation therapy (RT) is more challenging. Serum PSA levels slowly decrease after completing RT for localized prostate cancer. The nadir serum PSA level is expected at 18 months or more posttreatment (2). While lower nadir PSA levels have better prognosis, there is no absolute or relative PSA nadir that is associated with definitive treatment success. It is therefore necessary to define recurrence relative to the PSA nadir for each individual patient. The American Society for Radiation Oncology (ASTRO) defines biochemical relapse as a serum PSA 2 ng/mL greater than the nadir PSA level (3). This measurement should be repeated to confirm the level and to exclude a PSA bounce. PSA bounce is a phenomenon wherein the serum PSA level rises transiently between 12 and 18 months after radiation treatment but is not associated with relapse or failure of the primary treatment (4).

MANAGEMENT OF PSA INCREASE

While biochemical recurrence is common, it is not necessarily predictive of development of metastatic disease or of cancer-specific mortality. Initial management of PSA increase should include serial PSA monitoring, evaluation for local and distant disease with imaging, and prostate bed or other biopsies as guided by imaging results. Many patents will have biochemical evidence of disease with an indolent course. Thus, risk stratification is important in counseling patients in these clinical situations. PSA doubling time and Gleason score have been demonstrated to be independent predictors of prognosis in the event of biochemical relapse. Individuals with a PSA doubling time greater than 12 to 15 months are more likely to have an indolent course, whereas those with PSA doubling times less than 3 months are at 20-fold higher risk of cancer-related death compared to those with longer doubling times. The Gleason score from initial diagnosis or prostatectomy remains a significant prognostic factor in biochemical relapse. Men with biochemical relapse and Gleason scores of less than 7 are at lower risk of developing metastatic disease and cancer-related death compared to those with scores of 7 to 10 (5,6). Additionally, it is important to take into account the age of the patient, comorbid medical conditions, and personal preferences when counseling regarding management of biochemical recurrence.

SALVAGE THERAPY AFTER RADICAL PROSTATECTOMY

In men with biochemical relapse after radical prostatectomy and no evidence of metastatic disease, consideration of salvage external beam radiation therapy (EBRT) is recommended. While there are no randomized studies of salvage EBRT versus observation, several retrospective studies support prolonged disease-free survival in patients who received salvage EBRT (7). For men with particularly high-risk disease at the time of initial surgery—Gleason score 8 or more, seminal vesicle invasion, preoperative PSA more than 20—it is worth considering EBRT with concurrent androgen deprivation therapy (ADT) for 6 months (8). ADT, is appropriate for men who are not candidates for, or do not want, salvage EBRT but warrant treatment. Alternately, in older men or men with severe comorbidities, observation is a reasonable option.

SALVAGE THERAPY AFTER DEFINITIVE RADIATION THERAPY

There are several options for local salvage therapy of biochemical relapse after definitive RT, including radical prostatectomy, cryotherapy, and brachytherapy. No prospective clinical trials have evaluated local salvage therapies versus observation, and thus, biopsy-proven local recurrence and selection of appropriate patients is critical when considering local salvage therapy after definitive RT. Men who had earlier stage, lower risk disease (T1 or T2, Gleason score less than 8) at the time of diagnosis have been shown to have better outcomes relative to men with high-risk disease at diagnosis (9). Additionally, men with serum PSA levels less than 10 ng/mL at the time of salvage surgery have better outcomes (10). Men with high-risk disease at the time of initial diagnosis are less likely to benefit from local salvage therapies for treatment of biochemical relapse after RT, as they are more likely to progress to systemic disease. Such patients do better with ADT or observation. In appropriately selected men with biochemical relapse after definitive RT who have a life expectancy of more than 10 years, it is reasonable to consider salvage radical prostatectomy (11). Cryotherapy and brachytherapy are also reasonable salvage options.

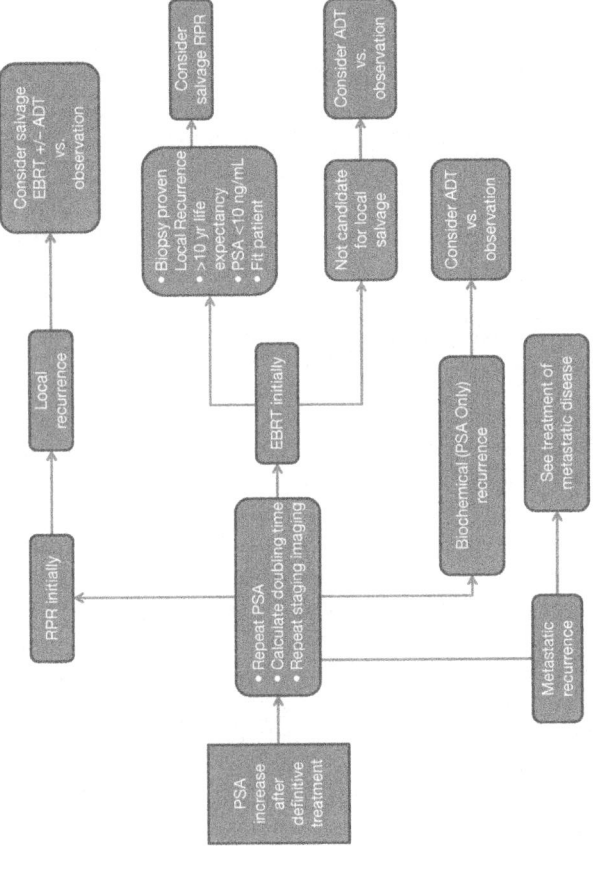

Figure 3.1 Choices of therapy following recurrence after local therapy.

ADT, androgen deprivation therapy; EBRT, external beam radiation therapy; PSA, prostate-specific antigen; RPR, radical retroperitoneal prostatectomy.

However, these are less well studied than salvage radical prostatectomy. Given the lack of clinical evidence comparing local salvage therapies to one another or to observation, it is important to take into account available expertise and experience when discussing salvage treatment options with patients (Figure 3.1).

> **KEY POINTS**
>
> - Biochemical recurrence is common and does not necessarily predict development of metastatic disease or cancer-specific mortality.
> - Risk stratification is important in counseling patients in these clinical situations. PSA doubling time and Gleason score are independent predictors of prognosis in the event of biochemical relapse.
> - Salvage therapy with EBRT, surgery, or ADT may be appropriate, depending on the initial modality of treatment and the patient's clinical factors.

REFERENCES

1. Cookson MS, Aus G, Burnett AL, et al. Variation in the definition of biochemical recurrence in patients treated for localized prostate cancer: the American Urological Association Prostate Guidelines for Localized Prostate Cancer Update Panel report and recommendations for a standard in the reporting of surgical outcomes. *J Urol.* 2007;177(2):540-545.
2. Crook JM, Choan E, Perry GA, et al. Serum prostate-specific antigen profile following radiotherapy for prostate cancer: implications for patterns of failure and definition of cure. *Urology.* 1998;51(4):566-572.
3. Roach M 3rd, Hanks G, Thames H Jr., et al. Defining biochemical failure following radiotherapy with or without hormonal therapy in men with clinically localized prostate cancer: recommendations of the RTOG-ASTRO Phoenix Consensus Conference. *Int J Radiat Oncol Biol Phys.* 2006;65(4):965-974.
4. Pickles T, British Columbia Cancer Agency Prostate Cohort Outcomes Initiative. Prostate-specific antigen (PSA) bounce and other fluctuations: which biochemical relapse definition is least prone to PSA false calls? An analysis of 2,030 men treated for prostate cancer with external beam or brachytherapy with or

without adjuvant androgen deprivation therapy. *Int J Radiat Oncol Biol Phys.* 2006;64(5):1355-1359.
5. Antonarakis ES, Feng Z, Trock BJ, et al. The natural history of metastatic progression in men with prostate-specific antigen recurrence after radical prostatectomy: long-term follow-up. *BJU Int.* 2012;109(1):32-39.
6. Zhou P, Chen MH, McLeod D, et al. Predictors of prostate cancer-specific mortality after radical prostatectomy or radiation therapy. *J Clin Oncol.* 2005;23(28):6992-6998.
7. Valicenti RK, Thompson I Jr, Albertsen P, et al. Adjuvant and salvage radiation therapy after prostatectomy: American Society for Radiation Oncology/American Urological Association guidelines. *Int J Radiat Oncol Biol Phys.* 2013;86(5):822-828.
8. Carrie C, Hasbini A, de Laroche G, et al. Salvage radiotherapy with or without short-term hormone therapy for a rising prostate-specific antigen concentration after radical prostatectomy (GETUG-AFU 16): a randomised, multicentre, open-label phase 3 trial. *Lancet Oncol.* 2016;17(6):747-756.
9. Nguyen PL, D'Amico AV, Lee AK, Suh WW. Patient selection, cancer control, and complications after salvage local therapy for postradiation prostate-specific antigen failure: a systematic review of the literature. *Cancer.* 2007;110(7):1417-1428.
10. Tiguert R, Rigaud J, Lacombe L, et al. Neoadjuvant hormone therapy before salvage radiotherapy for an increasing post-radical prostatectomy serum prostate specific antigen level. *J Urol.* 2003;170(2 Pt 1):447-450.
11. Chade DC, Eastham J, Graefen M, et al. Cancer control and functional outcomes of salvage radical prostatectomy for radiation-recurrent prostate cancer: a systematic review of the literature. *Eur Urol.* 2012;61(5):961-971.

Intermittent Androgen Ablation in Biochemical Relapse of Early Stage Prostate Cancer

Chitra Balasundaram and Teresa Gray Hayes

DEFINITION OF BIOCHEMICAL RELAPSE

The definition of biochemical relapse (BCR) depends on the type of definitive treatment the patient received for initial management of localized prostate cancer. Since all prostatic tissue is removed by radical prostatectomy (RP), the prostate-specific antigen (PSA) levels should be undetectable by 4 weeks after RP, as the half-life of PSA is about 3 days. If the PSA fails to nadir after RP, this indicates residual prostate tissue either locally or as distant metastases, and is called biochemical failure. The most widely accepted definition of BCR after RP is that of the American Urological Association (AUA) and is defined as a serum PSA greater than 0.2 ng/mL, which is confirmed by a second determination with a PSA of greater than 0.2 ng/mL. In contrast to RP, with radiation treatment, there is still some residual prostatic tissue and the PSA slowly nadirs over a period of 18 months. Also, in intermediate and high-risk disease, after completion of radiation treatment short- or long-term androgen deprivation therapy (ADT) is used, and this can confound the PSA values. The Phoenix criteria are currently used to determine BCR after radiation treatment. A PSA rise of 2 ng/mL or more above the nadir PSA is considered BCR after external beam radiation therapy (EBRT), regardless of whether or not a patient receives short-term or long-term ADT. This is generally confirmed by a repeat measurement of PSA in 3 to 6 months.

INCIDENCE OF BCR

About 40% of men diagnosed with prostate cancer undergo RP as their primary cancer therapy. About one-third of men undergoing RP will develop detectable PSA levels (BCR) within 10 years after the operation. The BCR rate after EBRT is 40% to 60%. If biochemical failure or recurrence goes untreated, about one-third of patients will develop detectable metastatic disease within 8 years after RP (1). After EBRT, about one-fourth of patients will develop detectable metastatic disease within 5 years and the median time to prostate cancer–specific mortality is 10 years (2).

TREATMENT OF BCR

The approach to treatment of BCR varies, as development of BCR does not necessarily predict development of metastases, and many patients may have indolent disease that does not require treatment. The decision to start systemic therapy, that is ADT, is influenced by a number of prognostic factors, namely age, underlying comorbidities, psychosocial factors/patient anxiety, tumor characteristics at time of initial definitive therapy (Gleason's score, stage, PSA level, margin status), absolute PSA level at the time of BCR, and PSA doubling time (PSADT). The most important factors are a short PSADT and high Gleason's score (3,4).

- If the PSADT is greater than 12 months, and the patient is elderly, observation may be considered.
- If there is no evidence of distant metastatic disease clinically or radiographically, then some patients (stage T1–T2, N0 or NX, PSA now < 10 ng/mL, life expectancy > 10 years) are candidates for salvage local treatment, which may include radiation after failed RP or cryosurgery after failed EBRT.
- ADT is considered when the risk of systemic disease is high based on the pathologic and clinical factors, and hence not treatable by salvage local therapy; or if the patient is not a candidate for local treatment due to underlying comorbidities or patient preference.

ANDROGEN DEPRIVATION THERAPY

Once the decision to give ADT for treatment for BCR has been made, the timing of when to start ADT presents a therapeutic dilemma. There is no consensus to the definition of early ADT versus late ADT (i.e., at what PSA level should ADT be initiated). Early ADT may prevent progression and hence may prolong survival, though there is no clear evidence of survival advantage by this approach. Delayed ADT until clinically overt metastasis is seen may be advocated, as ADT is associated with significant side effects and there is no clear survival advantage (5,6). Hence, treatment should be individualized until more evidence is available to support one approach over the other. Earlier systemic therapy is recommended for younger age, high grade disease (Gleason's score of 8–10), and shorter PSADT of less than 10 to 12 months.

Options for ADT include complete androgen blockade versus monotherapy. There are no randomized trials comparing complete androgen blockade (Gonadotropin-releasing hormone [GnRH] analogue + antiandrogen) to either GnRH or orchiectomy alone. Most of the studies looking at treatment of BCR with ADT used complete androgen blockade (5).

INTERMITTENT VERSUS CONTINUOUS ADT

Long-term ADT is associated with significant side effects including but not restricted to loss of libido and potency, hot flashes, and loss of bone and muscle mass. The rationale for trying intermittent (as opposed to continuous) ADT is 2-fold: to decrease these side effects and hence improve quality of life (QOL); and theoretically, continuous ADT may facilitate progression from androgen dependence (castrate-sensitive disease) to androgen independence (castrate-resistant disease), which may be delayed by use of intermittent ADT.

Intermittent ADT involves use of cyclic ADT: ADT is initiated and continued till serum PSA is lowered to a certain predefined level. This is followed by temporary withdrawal of ADT. Another cycle of ADT is restarted when serum PSA increases to a predefined level (usually 2.5–20 ng/mL) or serum testosterone is no longer at castrate levels (>20–50 ng/mL). Patients who are on intermittent ADT may be off ADT 35% to 50% of the time.

The most extensive data for intermittent androgen deprivation (IAD) come from the Canadian led PR 7 trial (7). In this international randomized phase 3 trial, 1,386 men with a rising PSA greater than 3 ng/mL after RT were randomized to receive either IAD or continuous ADT. Patients assigned to IAD received therapy for 8 months and treatment was restarted when the serum PSA reached greater than 10 ng/mL off treatment. The primary end point was overall survival. The study was designed to show noninferiority. At a median follow-up of 6.9 years, the intermittent approach was noninferior to the continuous approach with respect to overall survival (median 8.8 vs. 9.1 years, hazard ratio [HR] 1.02, 95% confidence interval [CI] 0.86–1.21). Men treated with IAD had more prostate cancer–related deaths (120 out of 690 patients) than in the continuous ADT arm (94 of 696 patients) but this was balanced by more non-prostate-cancer-related deaths in the continuous ADT arm. QOL analyses showed statistically significant modest benefits in the IAD group when it came to symptoms of loss of libido, urinary symptoms, and hot flashes. However, only 214 out of 1,386 (15%) patients had died when the results of the trial were analyzed and longer follow-up may be required for disease-specific deaths to outbalance deaths by other causes. An unplanned Cox regression analysis showed that men with a Gleason's score greater than 7 had a 14-month increased survival with continuous ADT (8.0 years) as compared to IAD (6.8 years). Hence, IAD should be offered to patients only after explaining the full risks of potential harm versus benefits from improved QOL.

Currently, the American Society of Clinical Oncology (ASCO) recommends continuous ADT over IAD, due to lack of sufficient long-term evidence (5). However, National Comprehensive Cancer Network guidelines recommend consideration of intermittent androgen deprivation (8).

KEY POINTS

- Systemic therapy/ADT for BCR in early stage prostate cancer is considered in patients who are thought to be at high risk for disseminated disease (despite absence

(continued)

(continued)

> of clinical or radiographic evidence of the same), or those who are not candidates for salvage local therapy due to patient preference or underlying comorbidities.
> - Options for ADT include continuous versus intermittent ADT. The current body of evidence is not sufficient to support intermittent over continuous ADT.
> - Intermittent ADT may be offered to certain patients, after counseling them about the risks of decreased survival versus the benefits of better QOL.

REFERENCES

1. Antonarakis ES, Feng Z, Trock BJ, et al. The natural history of metastatic progression in men with prostate-specific antigen recurrence after radical prostatectomy: long-term follow-up. *BJU Int.* 2012;109(1):32-39.
2. Zumsteg ZS, Spratt DE, Romesser PB, et al. The natural history and predictors of outcome following biochemical relapse in the dose escalation era for prostate cancer patients undergoing definitive external beam radiotherapy. *Eur Urol.* 2015;67(6):1009-1016.
3. Zhou P, Chen MH, McLeod D, et al. Predictors of prostate cancer-specific mortality after radical prostatectomy or radiation therapy. *J Clin Oncol.* 2005;23(28):6992-6998.
4. D'Amico AV, Moul JW, Carroll PR, et al. Surrogate end point for prostate cancer-specific mortality after radical prostatectomy or radiation therapy. *J Natl Cancer Inst.* 2003;95(18):1376-1383.
5. Loblaw DA, Virgo KS, Nam R, et al. Initial hormonal management of androgen-sensitive metastatic, recurrent, or progressive prostate cancer: 2006 update of an American Society of Clinical Oncology practice guideline. *J Clin Oncol.* 2007;25(12):1596-1605.
6. Garcia-Albeniz X, Chan JM, Paciorek AT, et al. Immediate versus deferred initiation of androgen deprivation therapy in prostate cancer patients with PSA-only relapse [abstract]. American Society of Clinical Oncology meeting. *J Clin Oncol.* 2014; 32(suppl):5s. Abstract 5003.
7. Crook JM, O'Callaghan CJ, Duncan G, et al. Intermittent androgen suppression for rising PSA level after radiotherapy. *N Engl J Med.* 2012;367(10):895-903.
8. Prostate Cancer Guidelines Version 3.2016. NCCN Clinical Practice Guidelines in Oncology (NCCN Guidelines®) for Prostate Cancer V.3.2016. © National Comprehensive Cancer Network, Inc. 2016.

Treatment of Therapy Complications   5

Pranav Dadhich and Jennifer Marie Taylor

INTRODUCTION

The management of prostate cancer has evolved rapidly over the last few decades. The focus of this section is on the complications associated with definitive treatment of the primary disease with surgery or radiation therapy (RT). Both of these modalities can have significant effects on urinary continence and erectile function. Generally, the functional side effects of surgery are immediate and improve with time, whereas the long-lasting side effects of RT can gradually worsen over time. A recent report of quality of life outcomes in men undergoing both primary modalities in the Prostate Cancer Outcomes Study (PCOS) indicate similar rates of urinary and erectile complaints at 15 years (1).

URINARY INCONTINENCE

Urinary incontinence can be seen after both prostatectomy and RT. The physical removal of the prostate gland and associated trauma invariably alter flow dynamics of the bladder outlet. Injury to the external urinary sphincter and loss of the constrictive effect created by the prostate and bladder neck paves the way for stress urinary incontinence (SUI). RT can alter the outlet through gradual fibrosis and potential for urethral stricture formation. Both surgery and RT can alter detrusor muscle function and lead to or unmask irritative voiding symptoms, such as urinary urgency and frequency.

Systematic reviews of postprostatectomy data have shown that the rates of SUI after surgery are highly variable and depend on many factors, both patient and surgeon related. The incidence of SUI has been reported to range from 7% to 40% after open surgery and 4% to 31% after robotic intervention (2). Irritative symptoms affect up to 25% or more of men who receive prostate RT, but long-term urinary irritative symptoms are less common, affecting 5% to 10% of men. Studies show that the rates of urethral scarring are quite close when comparing brachytherapy and external beam radiation therapy (EBRT). Current data show that stricture rates stand at 1.8% and 1.7%, respectively (3). Alongside strictures, bladder dysfunction has also been observed in patients receiving EBRT. Studies have shown that scatter radiation can reduce bladder filling capacity (4), which can impair bladder compliance and induce urinary frequency and hyperreflexia.

The irritative symptoms can often be managed with dietary and lifestyle modifications, followed by medical therapy such as anticholinergic agents. Stress incontinence can be mitigated with Kegel exercises and pelvic floor therapy. If stress incontinence persists beyond 12 months after surgery and is bothersome, surgical interventions are available, including urethral bulking agents, urethral sling placement, and artificial urinary sphincter prosthesis placement (5). In the case of posttherapy urethral stricture disease that affects a patient's emptying, surgical options include urethral dilation, endoscopic visual urethrotomy, or urethroplasty reconstructive surgery (6).

ERECTILE DYSFUNCTION

One of the biggest concerns for men after prostatectomy is erectile dysfunction. The prostate facilitates ejaculation, removing the ability for emission of seminal fluid after surgery. Additionally, the cavernosal nerves that provide autonomic regulation of erections travel in the fascial layers on the lateral aspect of the prostate gland and are at risk of injury with surgery or any energy delivery modality such as radiation or ablation. Significant data have been reported on the predictors and mechanisms of erectile dysfunction; however, vast variation exists and definitive conclusions are hard to reach. An extensive literature review indicates that rates of complete erectile dysfunction after surgery (refractory to all medical therapy) range from 26% to 100% and rates of partial erectile dysfunction range from 16% to 48% (7). Data demonstrate that it can take on average up to 24 months to fully recover erectile function after surgery, and RT can cause continued fibrosis and loss of function with time. Some recent data have shown that patients have reported a greater magnitude of erectile dysfunction with EBRT compared to brachytherapy (8), but this subject continues to warrant further investigation.

Surgical technique has undergone refinements with a better understanding of preservation of the neurovascular bundle. During nerve sparing surgery, emphasis is placed on careful dissection and maintenance of three neurologic focal points: proximal neurovascular plate, predominant neurovascular bundle, and accessory neural pathways (9). Literature shows that in major academic centers, erectile function recovery occurs at rates ranging from 60% to 85%. Currently, many surgeons have instituted programs of postsurgical penile rehabilitation, to include use of phosphodiesterase type 5 (PDE-5) inhibitors and other methods, as a means of improving the time to recovery (10). Management of erectile dysfunction proceeds stepwise from oral medication (PDE-5 inhibitors), to intra-urethral medication and intra-cavernosal injections, and finally to penile prosthesis placement.

Impotence also remains an important pathological consequence of radiotherapy. Scatter radiation has potential to affect pelvic nerve bundles and diminish erectile function as well as to damage local tissue that is important in both erection and ejaculation.

KEY POINTS

- Treatment of prostate cancer can have significant effects on urinary continence and erectile function.
- The rates of urinary and erectile complaints are similar at 15 years after surgery and RT.
- Refined surgical and radiation techniques can minimize the frequency of side effects.
- Techniques are available to address symptoms of bladder and erectile dysfunction occurring after prostate cancer treatment.

REFERENCES

1. Resnick M, Koyama T, Fan K, et al. Long-term functional outcomes after treatment for localized prostate cancer. *NEJM.* 2013;368:436-445.
2. Ficarra V, Novara G, Rosen RC, et al. Systematic review and meta-analysis of studies reporting urinary continence recovery after robot-assisted radical prostatectomy. *Eur Urol.* 2012;62(3):405-417.
3. Khourdaji I, Parke J, Chennamsetty A, Burks F. Treatment of urethral strictures from irradiation and other nonsurgical forms of pelvic cancer treatment. *Adv Urol.* 2015;2015: Article ID 476390, 7 pages.
4. Méndez-Rubio S, Salinas-Casado J, Vírseda-Chamorro M, et al. Long-term adverse effects on bladder filling phase in males submitted to the pelvic radiotherapy. *Arch Esp Urol.* 2015;68(7):609-614.
5. Léon P, Chartier-Kastler E, Rouprêt M, et al. Long-term functional outcomes after artificial urinary sphincter implantation in men with stress urinary incontinence. *BJU Int.* 2015;115(6):951-957.
6. LaBossiere JR, Cheung D, Rourke K. Endoscopic treatment of vesicourethral stenosis after radical prostatectomy: outcomes and predictors of success. *J Urol.* 2016;195(5):1495-1500.
7. Burnett AL, Aus G, Canby-Hagino ED, et al. American Urological Association Prostate Cancer Guideline Update Panel. Erectile function outcome reporting after clinically localized prostate cancer treatment. *J Urol.* 2007;178(2):597-601.
8. Putora PM, Engeler D, Haile SR, et al. Erectile function following brachytherapy, external beam radiotherapy, or radical prostatectomy in prostate cancer patients. *Strahlenther Onkol.* 2016;192(3):182-189.
9. Tewari A, Takenaka A, Mtui E, et al. The proximal neurovascular plate and the tri-zonal neural architecture around the prostate gland: importance in the athermal robotic technique of nerve-sparing prostatectomy. *BJU Int.* 2006;98(2):314-323.
10. Burnett AL. Current rehabilitation strategy: clinical evidence for erection recovery after radical prostatectomy. *Transl Androl Urol.* 2013;2(1):24-31.

Early Stage Prostate Cancer: Controversies in Management   6

Jianbo Wang and Teresa Gray Hayes

INTRODUCTION

Prostate cancer is the second most common type of cancer in men around the world (1). It is a clinically heterogeneous disease, and the clinical course and aggressiveness of prostate cancer varies widely from patient to patient. This heterogeneity makes it difficult to implement evidence-based clinical practice guidelines to every single patient. As such, controversy has arisen over the management of prostate cancer. This chapter discusses the controversies surrounding prostate cancer screening, treatment strategies of localized prostate cancer, androgen deprivation treatment, and the role of proton therapy.

PROSTATE CANCER SCREENING

Case 1: A 48-year-old African American male presents for consultation about prostate cancer screening. One of his brothers was diagnosed with prostate cancer at the age of 60 years.

Question 1: Should he undergo prostate cancer screening?
Prostate cancer often grows slowly. The 5-year survival of patients with prostate cancer confined within the prostate and local spread is about 100% versus 29.3% for patients with distant metastasis (2). It seems reasonable that prostate cancer screening would be able to reduce morbidity and mortality in the subset of asymptomatic patients with aggressive localized prostate cancer. Unfortunately, prostate cancer screening is not well supported by data from randomized studies.

Limitation in the design and differing results of randomized trials are to blame for lack of supportive data for screening.

Two large randomized trials were done to evaluate the effectiveness of prostate cancer screening. The European Randomized Study of Screening for Prostate Cancer (ERSPC) randomized 182,160 men between the ages of 50 and 74 to prostate-specific antigen (PSA) screening. Follow-up was truncated at 13 years for the 162,243 men in a prespecified core group between the ages of 55 and 69. The absolute rates of prostate cancer mortality were 0.43 versus 0.54 per 1,000 person-years. Forty-eight additional patients needed to be diagnosed to prevent one prostate cancer death. Although there are factors in this trial that biased results toward effects or no effects, the absolute benefit of prostate cancer screening was low (3).

In the U.S. Prostate, Lung, Colorectal and Ovarian Cancer (PLCO) Screening Trial, 76,693 men between the ages of 55 and 74 were randomly assigned to annual screening with PSA and digital rectal examination (DRE) or to usual care. After 7 years of follow-up and longer-term follow-up, there was no reduction in the primary outcome of prostate cancer (4). The negative results of the PLCO trial may be confounded by the high rate of PSA testing in the control arm, a higher PSA cutoff for biopsy, and the substantial proportion of men with abnormal PSA and/or DRE results who had not undergone biopsy within 3 years following the positive screen.

Furthermore, a 2010 meta-analysis summarized results from six randomized trials. Screening with PSA with or without DRE compared to no screening did not reduce death from prostate cancer (5). In 2011, a Cochrane meta-analysis had similar findings (6). However, screening did significantly increase the probability of cancer diagnosis.

In addition to conflicting results regarding the efficacy of prostate cancer screening as shown in randomized trials, prostate cancer screening is associated with significant risks of biopsy, overdiagnosis, and treatment. However, once prostate cancer has advanced far enough to cause symptoms, it is generally no longer localized and is therefore incurable. As a result, it is important to discuss potential benefits and risks of prostate cancer screening with patients. More importantly, involving patients in the shared decision-making process and using a decision-making aid have been proven to decrease screening rate, increase screening satisfaction, and decrease decision conflicts in systemic reviews and randomized trials (7,8).

TREATMENT OF LOCALIZED PROSTATE CANCER

Case 2: A 55-year-old male was recently found to have a PSA of 8 ng/mL. No abnormality was detected on DRE. Prostate biopsies showed two positive biopsy cores with less than 50% involvement in any one core.

Question 2: What kind of treatment options can be offered to this patient?

Due to widely used prostate cancer screening, many men were diagnosed with clinically localized prostate cancer. The biggest concern is if the diagnosed prostate cancer is clinically significant enough to warrant medical treatment. Besides, selection for optimal treatment for the individual patient is often complicated and controversial due to underlying tumor heterogeneity. The treatment options include active surveillance, radiation therapy, and prostatectomy. In general, treatment planning needs to take into account the patient's life expectancy, comorbidities, risk stratification of cancer, and preference. Based on baseline PSA, Gleason score, and the extent of prostate involvement, patients can be divided into very-low-, low-, intermediate-, high-, and very-high-risk groups. For patients with very-low-risk cancer and life expectancy less than 20 years, active surveillance is preferred. In patients with low-risk prostate cancer and life expectancy greater than 10 years, definitive therapy (radiation and prostatectomy) or active surveillance is acceptable (9,10). For patients with intermediate-, high-, and very-high-risk prostate cancer, definitive treatment (radical prostatectomy or radiation) is recommended. Side effects are different for each treatment. Radiation may be associated with gastrointestinal symptoms, urinary symptoms, and erectile dysfunction. Prostatectomy can result in urinary incontinence and erectile dysfunction. Although active surveillance does not cause the aforementioned side effects, it does induce significant stress and anxiety. As a result, patients on active surveillance often end up getting radiation therapy or prostatectomy. Oftentimes, the choice of treatment is left up to the discretion of clinicians in collaboration with patients.

RADIATION TREATMENT: PROTON THERAPY

Case 3: A 75-year-old male presented with newly diagnosed prostate cancer. He has disease limited to one lobe of the prostate, a serum PSA 7 ng/mL, and a Gleason score of 4.

Question 3: Is this patient a candidate for proton therapy?
Because of the unique physical properties of heavy particles, a proton beam results in the majority of the energy being deposited at the end of a linear track, reducing the dose to normal tissues. Although many proton treatment centers have opened in recent years, there are no randomized trials that compare proton beam therapy with photon beam therapy or brachytherapy in men with clinically localized prostate cancer. A systematic review of the available evidence from the American Society for Radiation Oncology (ASTRO) on efficacy and toxicity concluded that outcomes were similar with proton beam therapy and intensity-modulated radiation therapy (IMRT), but did not demonstrate an advantage for the proton beam approach (11).

As mentioned earlier, controversy in management of prostate cancer stems from the underlying heterogeneity. Hopefully, these controversies might be resolved by tailoring treatment to the individual's genetic makeup in the era of personalized oncology.

KEY POINTS

- Screening for prostate cancer carries the risk of possible overdiagnosis and overtreatment. As a result, it is important to discuss potential benefits and risks of prostate cancer screening with patients.
- Treatment of localized prostate cancer should be tailored to the factors in the individual patient including aggressiveness of the cancer, cancer stage, and life expectancy.

REFERENCES

1. International Agency for Research on Cancer. Cancer fact sheets: Prostate cancer. http://gco.iarc.fr/today/fact-sheets-cancers?cancer=19&type=0&sex=1. Accessed April 5, 2017.
2. Howlader N, Noone AM, Krapcho M, et al. SEER cancer statistics review, 1975-2013, Bethesda, MD: National Cancer Institute. http://seer.cancer.gov/csr/1975_2013/. Accessed April 5, 2017.
3. Schröder FH, Hugosson J, Roobol MJ, et al. Screening and prostate-cancer mortality in a randomized European study. *N Engl J Med.* 2009;360(13):1320-1328.
4. Andriole GL, Crawford ED, Grubb RL, et al. Mortality results from a randomized prostate-cancer screening trial. *N Engl J Med.* 2009;360(13):1310-1319.
5. Djulbegovic M, Beyth RJ, Neuberger MM, et al. Screening for prostate cancer: systematic review and meta-analysis of randomised controlled trials. *BMJ.* 2010;341:c4543.
6. Ilic D, O'Connor D, Green S, Wilt TJ. Screening for prostate cancer: an updated Cochrane systematic review. *BJU Int.* 2011;107(6):882-891.
7. Volk RJ, Hawley ST, Kneuper S, et al. Trials of decision aids for prostate cancer screening: a systematic review. *Am J Prev Med.* 2007;33(5):428-434.
8. Taylor KL, Williams RM, Davis K, et al. Decision making in prostate cancer screening using decision aids vs usual care: a randomized clinical trial. *JAMA Intern Med.* 2013;173(18):1704-1712.
9. Mason MD, Parulekar WR, Sydes MR, et al. Final report of the Intergroup Randomized Study of Combined Androgen-Deprivation Therapy plus radiotherapy versus androgen-deprivation therapy alone in locally advanced prostate cancer. *J Clin Oncol.* 2015;33(19):2143-2150.
10. Wilt TJ, Brawer MK, Jones KM, et al. Radical prostatectomy versus observation for localized prostate cancer. *N Engl J Med.* 2012;367(3):203-213.
11. Allen AM, Pawlicki T, Dong L, et al. An evidence based review of proton beam therapy: the report of ASTRO's emerging technology committee. *Radiother Oncol.* 2012;103(1):8-11.

Early Stage Prostate Cancer Survivorship Challenges   7

Andrew Jackson and Teresa Gray Hayes

Prostate cancer is the second most common cancer in men, and long-term survival is common. It is important that patients continue to receive comprehensive care after completion of active therapy for their early stage prostate cancer. Care for cancer survivors is most effective when conducted in coordination between cancer specialists and primary care physicians. Studies have indicated that primary physicians are nine times more likely to counsel patients and actively participate in survivorship care when they have received a written care plan for the treating specialist. Effective survivorship care is focused in three areas: overall or general health, screening for recurrence or secondary cancers, and identification and management of treatment related side effects.

As men with early stage prostate cancer move from active treatment to surveillance and survivorship, it is important for physicians to talk with them about general health and the components of a healthy lifestyle. This counseling should focus on maintaining a healthy diet, weight management, continuing physical exercise, limiting alcohol intake, and avoiding or eliminating tobacco use. Additional topics of discussion should include optimal management of comorbid medical conditions and health maintenance including routine cancer screenings. Prostate cancer survivors, particularly those who have received androgen deprivation therapy (ADT), are at higher risk of developing hypertension, osteoporosis, dyslipidemia, and diabetes and should be screened by their primary care physicians for these conditions annually. Additionally, anemia is common in men during and after ADT.

Cancer survivors are often concerned about recurrence, and screening for recurrence is an essential part of survivorship care.

The American Cancer Society, American Society of Clinical Oncology, and National Comprehensive Cancer Network all recommend screening for prostate cancer recurrence with serum prostate-specific antigen (PSA) every 6 to 12 months during the first 5 years after treatment. After that time, annual serum PSA levels should be continued indefinitely. In addition to screening for prostate cancer recurrence, patients should also receive routine screening for secondary cancers, which may be related to treatment. It should be noted that men with prostate cancer treated with radiotherapy have a slightly increased risk for bladder and colorectal cancers, and thus particular attention should be given to early signs or symptoms of these cancers (1).

As a result of improving effectiveness of prostate cancer treatments, men may live for many years after treatment. Side effects of cancer treatment can be long-lived or even delayed in onset. Ongoing screening and management of bowel, urinary, bone, and sexual side effects are important. Additionally, evaluation of psychosocial effects of cancer and cancer treatment is important. Anxiety and depression are common among cancer patients, and these conditions can be effectively treated with medications and counseling. Many men report that the psychosocial effects of cancer treatment have a significant impact on their quality of life. Screening for and management of these conditions is an essential part of survivorship care.

KEY POINTS

- Coordination of posttreatment care is important between primary physicians and specialists.
- General health counseling is required.
- Screening for recurrence and secondary cancers should continue lifelong.
- Management of persistent and late side effects is essential.

REFERENCE

1. Skolarus TA, Wolf AMD, Erb NL, et al. American Cancer Society prostate cancer survivorship care guidelines. *CA: A Cancer Journal for Clinicians*. 2014;64:225-249.

MANAGEMENT OF ADVANCED
PROSTATE CANCER

Treatment of Metastatic Cancer: Hormonal Agents, Chemotherapy, Immune Modulation, and Radiopharmaceuticals 8

Jesus H. Hermosillo-Rodriguez and Teresa Gray Hayes

INTRODUCTION

Management of metastatic prostate cancer involves the sequential or combined use of multiple kinds of therapies. The goals are prolonging survival with reasonable side effect morbidity, and maintenance or improvement of the patient's quality of life. In this chapter, we focus on the effective disease-modifying therapies available. We mostly focus on adenocarcinoma histology, with brief mention of small cell cancer of the prostate.

CASTRATION SENSITIVE DISEASE

Androgen deprivation therapy (ADT), with the goal of lowering serum testosterone to castrate levels (<50 ng/dL), is the mainstay treatment for metastatic prostate cancer (1). For men whose only evidence of disease is an elevated PSA or for patients with asymptomatic low-volume metastases, the optimal timing of initiation of therapy is controversial, and will be discussed further in the controversies in management chapter. Although the duration of response to ADT is highly variable, initial objective tumor responses are around 80% to 90% with a median failure-free survival duration of 20 months and median overall survival (OS) of 42 months (2). There are several ways to prescribe ADT, and since they are considered equivalent in terms of effectiveness, choosing one of these

therapies is primarily based on patient preference, cost, and treatment availability. The typical antiandrogenic side effects of ADT include (3):
- Hot flashes, decreased body hair, and sexual dysfunction.
- Loss of lean body mass, increased body fat, and decreased muscle strength.
- Decreased bone mineral density.
- Gynecomastia and breast tenderness.
- Cardiovascular disease and insulin resistance.
- Emotional changes and cognitive impairment, although some of these could be accounted for by comorbidities, cancer stage, and other diseases that occur with aging.

The most currently used ADT are described below:
- **Surgical Orchiectomy** (1,3): Relatively simple and cost-effective with a rapid decline in testosterone. Useful when rapid response is a priority or when costs and adherence to therapy are a concern. The psychological effect is an important factor in patient preference and it may be ameliorated with placement of testicular prostheses or by performing a subcapsular orchiectomy.
- **Medical Castration** (1,3):
  - Gonadotropin releasing hormone (GnRH) agonists (e.g., leuprolide, goserelin, triptorelin): They bind to the GnRH receptors in the pituitary and cause an initial release of luteinizing hormone (LH), causing an early increase in testosterone, followed 1 week later by downregulation of GnRH receptors and decline in LH. Castration levels are reached within 3 to 4 weeks. The initial increase in testosterone can cause a "tumor flare," which might contribute to bone pain, urinary obstruction, or spinal cord compression. This can be prevented by bridging with antiandrogen therapy.
  - GnRH antagonists (Degarelix): They do not cause the initial testosterone level increase that GnRH agonists do and can achieve suppression of testosterone level within 3 days. However, injections have to be done monthly and local injection site reactions are reported more frequently.

- **Chemohormonal therapy** (1,2): Refers to the combination of ADT plus docetaxel. Traditionally docetaxel was reserved for the castration resistant setting. However, it might be beneficial in the castration sensitive patient. In the Systemic Therapy in Advancing or Metastatic Prostate Cancer: Evaluation for Drug Efficacy (STAMPEDE) trial, 1,184 patients with castration sensitive metastatic or high-risk locally-advanced disease were randomized to ADT plus 6 cycles of docetaxel and 10 mg prednisone daily or ADT alone. 61% of patients had metastatic disease. Docetaxel showed an OS benefit of 77 versus 67 months (hazard ratio [HR] 0.76, 95% confidence interval [CI] 0.63–0.91), and the benefit was seen particularly in metastatic disease (65 vs. 43 months). In the Chemohormonal Therapy versus Androgen Ablation Randomized Trial for Extensive Disease (CHAARTED) study, 790 patients with castration sensitive metastatic prostate cancer were randomized to 6 cycles of docetaxel and ADT or ADT alone. Chemohormonal therapy showed a benefit in median time to progression (20 vs. 12 months) and an OS benefit of 58 versus 44 months (HR 0.61, 95% CI 0.47–0.80). The benefit was particularly significant in the patients with high-volume disease (defined by visceral metastases and/or four or more bone metastases), with median survival of 49 versus 32 months (HR 0.61, 95% CI 0.52–0.72). Although there was a trend toward benefit, not enough events were seen in the low-volume disease group to reach a conclusion. An important limitation of this trial is that only 47% of patients in the ADT alone group received docetaxel at the time of castration resistance.

KEY POINTS FOR CASTRATION SENSITIVE METASTATIC PROSTATE CANCER

- The initial treatment for metastatic prostate cancer with low-volume disease (defined as no visceral metastases and <4 bone metastases) is ADT (Figure 8.1).
- Chemohormonal therapy combining ADT with docetaxel should be considered as initial treatment for high-volume disease.

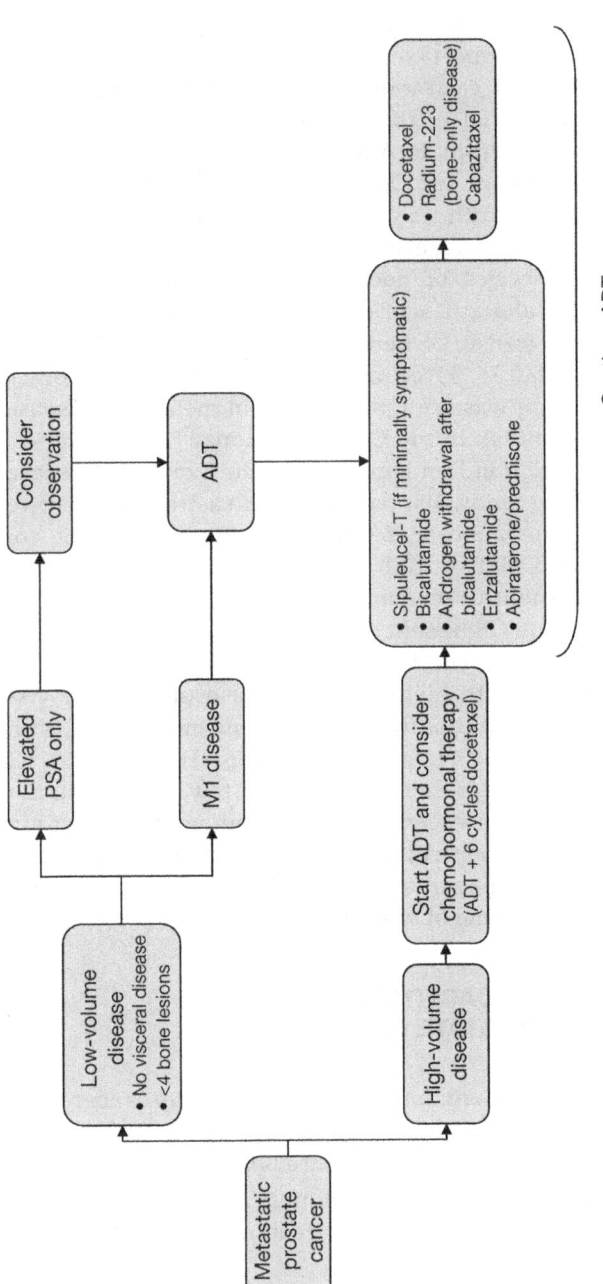

Figure 8.1 Treatment options for metastatic prostate cancer.

ADT, androgen deprivation therapy; PSA, prostate-specific antigen.

CASTRATION RESISTANT DISEASE

Eventually, prostate cancer progresses after administration of ADT, in spite of adequately depressed testosterone. This is labeled as castration resistant disease. Despite lack of randomized trial evidence, ADT is generally continued with subsequent therapies, due to the concern that discontinuation could result in a rise in testosterone and contribute to progression (3). Additional therapeutic options for castration resistant disease includes the following (see Figure 8.1):

- **First-generation antiandrogens (e.g., bicalutamide, nilutamide, flutamide)**: Although these agents have not been compared, bicalutamide is the most commonly used due to more favorable toxicity profile and suggestion of better efficacy. Besides antiandrogenic side effects, bicalutamide can rarely cause liver function abnormalities and diarrhea. Nilutamide can cause impaired dark adaptation and interstitial lung disease and flutamide has a risk of gastrointestinal side effects and significant liver toxicity.
- **Antiandrogen withdrawal** (3): After progression on a first-generation antiandrogen, metastatic prostate cancer may respond to withdrawal of the medication, evidenced by prostate-specific antigen (PSA) level. Significant PSA decline has been reported in around 15% to 20% of cases, though objective responses are rare. The waiting period for a withdrawal response is based on the half-life of the drug (3–6 weeks for bicalutamide).
- **Androgen synthesis inhibitors** (1,3): Although the majority of testosterone synthesis occurs in the testicles, the adrenal glands and tumor tissue also contribute to androgen synthesis. There are two main approved therapies to target androgen synthesis:
  - Abiraterone 1,000 mg/prednisone 5 mg oral bid: Potent irreversible inhibitor of 17 alpha-hydroxysteroid dehydrogenase (CYP17) in adrenal glands and tumor tissue.
    - Chemotherapy-naive setting: In a phase 3 trial of 1,088 patients, abiraterone/prednisone showed a radiographic progression-free survival of 16.5 versus 8.2 months compared to placebo/prednisone, and an OS benefit of 34.7 versus 30.3 months. Crossover occurred

in 44% of patients. There was a ≥50% PSA decline in 62% of patients, with objective responses of 36% and 61% stable disease.
- Post-docetaxel setting: In a randomized trial of the same comparison, the combination showed PSA progression time of 8.5 versus 6.6 months, and an OS benefit of 15.8 versus 11.2 months, with a ≥50% PSA response rate of almost 30% and objective responses of 14.8%.
- Besides antiandrogen side effects, there is inhibition of 17-alpha hydroxylase, which decreases cortisol production, and causes a rise in adrenocorticotropic hormone (ACTH) and increases mineralocorticoids. This can lead to hypertension, hypokalemia, and fluid retention, and is ameliorated by concurrent use of prednisone. Although less than with ketoconazole, there is a risk of adrenal insufficiency.
- Data is unclear of its benefit after progression on enzalutamide therapy, with some analysis suggesting limited activity.
- Ketoconazole 400 mg orally tid/hydrocortisone: Inhibits adrenal androgen synthesis in a less potent and specific way compared to abiraterone. It might retain a role in certain settings due to its lower cost. It requires a low gastric pH for maximum absorption so it should be taken on an empty stomach and without antacids. Most common side effects (besides antiandrogen side effects) include nausea, vomiting, rash, nail dystrophy, and hepatotoxicity. It can cause adrenal insufficiency so it is administered with hydrocortisone (20 mg in the morning and 10 mg in the evening). Medication interactions (like statins) should also be considered very carefully.
- **Enzalutamide 160 mg orally daily** (1): Enzalutamide is a pure androgen receptor competitive inhibitor, without agonistic properties like first-generation antiandrogens.
  - Chemotherapy-naive setting: The Multinational Phase 3, Randomized, Double-Blind, Placebo-Controlled Efficacy and Safety Study of Oral MDV3100 in Chemotherapy-Naive Patients With Progressive Metastatic Prostate Cancer Who Have Failed Androgen Deprivation Therapy (PREVAIL) trial, 1,717 patients were randomized to enzalutamide

versus placebo. Enzalutamide showed a radiographic progression-free survival at 12 months of 65% versus 14% (median not reached at 16.6 months), with a median OS benefit of 32.4 versus 30.2 months. PSA decline of ≥50% occurred in 78%, with objective responses of 59%. The main toxicity besides antiandrogen side effects was a small risk of seizures (<1%).

- Post-docetaxel setting: In the Safety and Efficacy Study of MDV3100 in Patients With Castration-Resistant Prostate Cancer Who Have Been Previously Treated With Docetaxel-based Chemotherapy (AFFIRM) trial, 1,199 patients were randomized to enzalutamide or placebo. Enzalutamide showed a time to PSA progression of 8.3 versus 3 months and an OS benefit of 18.4 versus 13.6 months (HR 0.63, 95% CI 0.53–0.75), with ≥50% PSA response of 54% and objective response of 29%.
- Data is unclear of its benefit after progression on abiraterone, with some retrospective analysis suggesting limited activity.

- **Immunotherapy—Sipuleucel-T** (1): A vaccine made out of the patient's dendritic cells that are removed by leukapheresis and exposed to prostatic acid phosphatase fused to granulocyte macrophage colony-stimulating factor. It is given every 2 weeks for 3 doses. In randomized trials in patients with minimally symptomatic castration resistant prostate cancer, sipuleucel-T showed an OS benefit of 25.8 versus 21.7 months compared to placebo. There were no responses or differences in disease progression.
- **Chemotherapy** (4): The first chemotherapy that was approved for castration resistant prostate cancer was mitoxantrone/prednisone, based on response in pain scores compared to placebo/prednisone. There was no benefit in OS, and the ≥50% PSA response was 33% compared to 22%. Because of these data, and the approval of newer therapies, its use has been limited. The only cytotoxic chemotherapy agents that have shown a significant OS benefit for patients with metastatic prostate cancer are taxanes.

- Docetaxel 75 mg/m^2 every 3 weeks with prednisone 5 mg oral bid: In the TAX 327 study in which 1,006 patients with castration resistant metastatic prostate cancer were randomized to 10 cycles of every 3 weeks docetaxel plus prednisone or every 3 weeks mitoxantrone plus prednisone, every 3-week docetaxel showed a median OS of 19.2 versus 16.3 months, with a 3-year survival of 18.6% versus 13.5%. There was a ≥50% PSA response of 45% and also higher rate of pain score improvement. Objective responses were 12% compared to 7%. There was a weekly docetaxel arm (30 mg/m^2 weekly for 5 of every 6 weeks) that had similar PSA response rate to 3-week docetaxel but did not have statistically significant improvement in pain scores compared to mitoxantrone, with an OS of 17.4 months.

- Docetaxel 50 mg/m^2 every 2 weeks with prednisone 5 mg oral bid (5): A multicenter trial of 346 patients with castration resistant prostate cancer were randomized to docetaxel 75 mg/m^2 every 3 weeks plus prednisone or docetaxel 50 mg/m^2 every 2 weeks plus prednisone. Granulocyte colony-stimulating factors were not given routinely. Two-week docetaxel showed a time to treatment failure (defined as disease progression, unacceptable toxic effects, death, or discontinuation of chemotherapy for any reason) of 5.6 months versus 4.9 months. The median number of cycles was 6 in each group and dose reductions were not significantly different. However, there were more delays in the 2-week group (10% vs. 5%). PSA response did not differ. Median OS was 19.5 months in the 2-week group versus 17 months in the 3-week group. Patients in the 3-week group had higher rates of grade 3 to 4 neutropenia (53% vs. 36%) as well as febrile neutropenia (14% vs. 4%).

- Cabazitaxel 25 mg/m^2 every 3 weeks with prednisone 10 mg oral daily (1,4): 10 cycles of cabazitaxel/prednisone were compared to 10 cycles of mitoxantrone/prednisone in the TROPIC trial with 755 patients who had progressed on docetaxel. Median progression free survival was 2.8 versus 1.4 months, and median OS was 15.1 versus 12.7 months. The 2-year survival rate was 27% versus 16%. Cabazitaxel had a ≥50% PSA response rate of 39.2%, with an objective response rate of 14.4%. Grade ≥3 neutropenia was seen in 82% of patients on cabazitaxel, with 8% having febrile neutropenia. Diarrhea was noted in 47% of patients on cabazitaxel, with 6% being grade ≥3.

- **Bone-targeted Radiopharmaceuticals** (1): The two main types used are alpha particle and beta particle emitters. The advantage of alpha emitters is that their decay allows the deposition of high energy radiation over a shorter distance than with beta particle emitters, minimizing bone marrow toxicity. An important prerequisite for this agent is the presence of uptake on bone scan due to metastatic disease at the sites that correlate with pain.
  - Alpha particle emitters: Radium-223 is the only agent that has a proven OS benefit. The Alpharadin in Symptomatic Prostate Cancer (ALSYMPCA) trial enrolled 921 patients with castration resistant prostate cancer with two or more bone lesions and no visceral metastases who were not candidates for, or had progressed on, docetaxel. Subjects were randomized to best supportive care plus radium-223 (given once every 4 weeks for 6 cycles) or best supportive care plus placebo. Forty percent of patients had 20 or more bone lesions. Radium-223 showed a benefit in time to first symptomatic skeletal event (defined as first use of external beam radiation therapy for symptom relief, new pathologic fracture, spinal cord compression, or tumor-related orthopedic surgery) of 15.6 versus 9.8 months. OS was 14.9 versus 11.3 months. Grade 3 to 4 thrombocytopenia was 9% in patients who had received docetaxel previously (compared to 3%).
  - Beta particle emitters: Although they have not shown OS benefit, these isotopes have shown improvement in bone pain, with the risk of myelosuppression. Their use has been limited to patients with bone pain who are not candidates for other therapies. The most commonly used are Strontium-89 and Samarium-153.

KEY POINTS FOR CASTRATION RESISTANT DISEASE

- The best sequence of treatment for castration resistant prostate cancer is unknown, and decision should be made based on clinical scenario, toxicity profile, cost, treatment availability, and patient preference (see Figure 8.1).

- Docetaxel is the initial chemotherapy agent recommended, with cabazitaxel reserved for the second-line setting.
- Radium-223 is the only radiopharmaceutical that has shown an OS benefit.

SMALL CELL CANCER OF PROSTATE

This malignancy is thought to arise from neuroendocrine cells derived from totipotent stem cells in the prostate (6). It typically affects younger patients, and mixed histology is not infrequent. Like small cell lung cancer, it usually predicts an aggressive behavior with rapid growth and spread, and paraneoplastic syndromes have been reported. A clue that can suggest small cell prostate cancer is the lack of correlation of PSA level and disease burden or disease progression, which should trigger a biopsy. Despite lack of clinical trial evidence, treatment is recommended in similar fashion to small cell lung cancer, with concurrent chemoradiation for limited-stage disease and cisplatin or carboplatin-based combination for extensive-stage disease. Whether ADT is beneficial for this subtype is unclear, but seems reasonable for patients with mixed histology. Survival rates seem similar to small cell lung cancer.

KEY POINT FOR SMALL CELL CANCER OF PROSTATE

- Small cell prostate cancer should be treated similarly to small cell lung cancer with concurrent chemoradiation for limited stage disease and palliative platinum-based chemotherapy for extensive stage.

REFERENCES

1. Park JC, Eisenberger MA. Advances in the treatment of metastatic prostate cancer. *Mayo Clinic Proceedings*. 2015;90(12):1719-1733.
2. James ND, Sydes MR, Mason MD, et al. Docetaxel and/or zoledronic acid for hormone-naive prostate cancer: first overall survival results from STAMPEDE (NCT00268476) [abstract]. *J Clin Oncol*. 2015;33(Suppl), Abstract 5001.

3. Perlmutter MA, Lepor H. Androgen deprivation therapy in the treatment of advanced prostate cancer [abstract]. *Rev Urol,* 2007; 9(suppl 1), S3-S8.
4. Sundararajan S, Vogelzang N. Chemotherapy in the treatment of prostate cancer—the past, the present, and the future. *American J Hematol/Oncol.* 2014;10(6):14-21.
5. Kellokumpu-Lehtinen PL, Harmenberg U, Joensuu T, et al. 2-weekly versus 3-weekly docetaxel to treat castration-resistant advanced prostate cancer: a randomised, phase 3 trial. *Lancet Oncol.* 2013;14:117-124.
6. Yashi M, Terauchi F, Nujui A, et al. Small-cell neuroendocrine carcinoma as a variant form of prostate cancer recurrence: a case report and short literature review. *Urol Oncol.* 2006;24(4):313-317.

Intermittent Androgen Ablation in Metastatic Prostate Cancer   9

Abhishek Marballi and Teresa Gray Hayes

INTRODUCTION

The role of androgens in the growth of prostate cancer was demonstrated by Huggins in 1941. This led the way for use of androgen deprivation therapy (ADT), which is now the backbone of systemic therapy for metastatic prostate cancer. Since prostate cancer is driven by androgen receptor signaling, ADT lowers testosterone levels into a castrate range, resulting in a decrease in prostate-specific antigen (PSA), which is driven by androgen receptor signaling.

PATHOPHYSIOLOGY

Androgen production takes place mainly in the testes, with a small contribution from the adrenal glands. The hypothalamus secretes gonadotropin releasing hormone (GnRH), which stimulates the anterior pituitary gland to release luteinizing hormone (LH) and follicle stimulating hormone (FSH). LH then circulates to Leydig cells in the testes, leading to the production of testosterone. Testosterone then goes to prostate epithelial cells, where it is converted into dihydrotestosterone (DHT) by the enzyme 5-alpha reductase. DHT binds with the androgen receptor and induces transcription of proteins necessary for function and development of the prostate. Androgens produced by the adrenal glands are androstenedione and dehydroepiandrosterone. These are released under the stimulation of adrenocorticotropic hormone (ACTH), which is secreted by the pituitary gland. The adrenal androgens play a role in the development of castrate resistant prostate cancer.

ANDROGEN DEPRIVATION THERAPY

ADT can be applied by surgical bilateral orchiectomy or medical castration. Target testosterone levels less than 50 ng/dL are used in most clinical studies and treatment protocols. Surgical bilateral orchiectomy can rapidly achieve testosterone levels less than 20 ng/dL. This method is cost saving, offers potentially fewer injections and clinic visits, and is equally as effective as medical castration in controlling prostate cancer. Interestingly, a study comparing GnRH agonists to orchiectomy in 3,295 men with prostate cancer selected from the Surveillance, Epidemiology, and End Results (SEER) database suggested that patients treated with GnRH analogs were at higher risk for fractures, peripheral arterial disease, venous thromboembolism, cardiac related complications, and diabetes mellitus ($P<.01$ for all) compared with orchiectomy (1). Despite this, medical castration is much more frequently used than surgical orchiectomy in North America. With medical castration, psychological issues of surgical castration can be avoided. This method is reversible and can be used to ameliorate hypogonadal symptoms. Agents that can be used for medical castration are GnRH agonists (leuprolide, goserelin, buserelin), GnRH antagonists (degarelix), androgen receptor blockers (bicalutamide, enzalutamide), and adrenal androgen synthesis inhibitors (abiraterone, ketoconazole).

INTERMITTENT VERSUS CONTINUOUS ANDROGEN DEPRIVATION THERAPY

ADT may increase the risk of osteoporosis, bone fractures, type 2 diabetes mellitus, myocardial infarction, stroke, erectile dysfunction, loss of libido, metabolic syndrome, weight gain, hot flashes, gynecomastia, fatigue, normocytic anemia, and alopecia (2,3). Multiple side effects from ADT can affect quality of life (QOL). Intermittent androgen deprivation therapy (IADT) involves alternating periods of medical castration and treatment free intervals to allow testosterone recovery. IADT is usually applied when there is a response to treatment with reintroduction of medical castration on progression of disease. The reason to consider IADT is to minimize adverse effects of treatment and improve QOL.

A study by Labarta et al randomized 49 patients to continuous androgen deprivation therapy (CADT) and 51 patients to IADT. Using a questionnaire, QOL between the two groups were compared. Results showed that the IADT group had significantly improved overall QOL as well as better scores for "sexual life" and "social partner support" (4). A randomized study by Mottet et al compared IADT and CADT in patients with metastatic prostate cancer. Patients with metastatic prostate cancer and prostate-specific antigen (PSA) of greater than 20 ng/mL received 6 months of induction ADT. If PSA level decreased below 4 ng/mL, they were then randomized to IADT or CADT. Results revealed a median overall survival of 52 months with CADT compared to 42 months with IADT, but this was not statistically significant ($P = .75$). Although scores regarding sexual function were significantly better in the IADT arm, most of the functional and symptom scales for QOL showed no significant differences between the two groups. However, there were significantly fewer treatment-emergent adverse events in the IADT group, with a lower incidence of hot flushes and headaches. This study concluded that IADT might be as safe as CADT in patients with metastatic prostate cancer and could be an option in highly responding and well-informed patients who have significant treatment induced side effects (5). In another study that compared IADT with CADT with regard to QOL, 852 men with metastatic prostate cancer received medical castration with goserelin. Patients whose PSA decreased to less than 10 ng/mL or by greater than 50% were randomized to IADT or CADT. QOL was monitored with a questionnaire. QOL was significantly better in the IADT arm with regard to physical capacity, activity limitation, and sexual functioning. Surprisingly, erectile dysfunction and depressed mood were significantly increased with IADT. There were no statistical differences in cardiovascular events, fractures, hot flushes, or night sweats (Table 9.1) (5–7).

A phase 3 noninferiority study by Hussain et al comparing IADT and CADT included 1,535 patients with metastatic prostate cancer. The coprimary objectives were to assess if IADT was noninferior to CADT in terms of survival, with 1.20 as the upper boundary of hazard ratio (HR), and whether there was any difference in QOL. Results revealed a median survival of 5.8 years with CADT and 5.1 years with IADT (HR 1.10 and confidence interval 0.99–1.23). There were no significant

Table 9.1 Comparison of Continuous Versus Intermittent Androgen Deprivation Therapy

Continuous ADT	Intermittent ADT
ADT continued without interruption	ADT held on response and reintroduced on progression
Median OS 5.8 y, trend toward better survival	Median OS 5.1 y, 20% greater risk of death cannot be ruled out
Worse sexual function	Relatively improved sexual function
Higher hot flushes and headaches	Lower hot flushes and headaches
Worse QOL in terms of physical capacity and activity limitation	Improved QOL in terms of physical capacity and activity limitation
Similar erectile dysfunction and mental health after mo 3	Better erectile dysfunction and mental health at mo 3
No difference in high-grade adverse events	No difference in high-grade adverse events

ADT, androgen deprivation therapy; OS, overall survival; QOL, quality of life.

differences in terms of treatment related high grade adverse events. However, IADT had significantly better erectile function and mental health at month 3, but not later. Since the confidence interval for survival exceeded the upper boundary of 1.2 for noninferiority, a 20% greater risk of death with IADT cannot be ruled out (7). Although there are a few studies concluding that IADT is as effective as CADT, these studies had suboptimal designs with mixed patient populations, poor noninferiority margin selection, and short follow-up times.

KEY POINTS

- The benefits of IADT compared to CADT in terms of QOL are modest at best, although statistically significant. It may not be meaningful to patients.
- Since IADT is not noninferior to CADT, CADT should be recommended in patients with metastatic prostate cancer.
- IADT can be considered in metastatic prostate cancer patients if they are highly responding and have uncontrolled significant treatment induced side effects.

REFERENCES

1. Sun M, Choueiri TK, Hamnvik OR, et al. Comparison of gonadotropin-releasing hormone agonists and orchiectomy: effects of androgen-deprivation therapy. *JAMA Oncol.* 2016 Apr;2(4):500–507. doi:10.1001/jamaoncol.2015.4917
2. Shahinian VB, Kuo YF, Freeman JL, et al. Risk of fracture after androgen deprivation for prostate cancer. *N Engl J Med.* 2005;352(2):154-164.
3. D'Amico AV1, Denham JW, Crook J, et al. Influence of androgen suppression therapy for prostate cancer on the frequency and timing of fatal myocardial infarctions. *J Clin Oncol.* 2007;25(17):2420-2425.
4. Sierra Labarta CR, Sánchez Zalabardo D, de Pablo Cárdenas A. Quality of life in patients diagnosed of prostate cancer treated with continuous androgen deprivation therapy vs. intermittent therapy. *An Sist Sanit Navar.* 2015;38(2):193-201.
5. Mottet N, Van Damme J, Loulidi S, et al. Intermittent hormonal therapy in the treatment of metastatic prostate cancer: a randomized trial. *BJU Int.* 2012;110:1262-1269.
6. Salonen AJ, Taari K, Ala-Opas M, et al. Advanced prostate cancer treated with intermittent or continuous androgen deprivation in the randomized Finn Prostate Study VII: quality of life and adverse effects. *Eur Urol.* 2013;63:111-120.
7. Hussain M, Tangen CM, Berry DL, et al. Intermittent versus continuous androgen deprivation in prostate cancer. *N Engl J Med.* 2013;368:1314-1325.

Bone Health and Use of Adjunctive Agents 10

Jesus H. Hermosillo-Rodriguez and Nicholas Mitsiades

An important issue in patients with prostate cancer is bone health, since both prostate cancer and its therapy can affect the bone. Typically, metastatic lesions from prostate cancer are osteoblastic. However, there is usually a significant osteolytic component, and pathologic fractures can occur. Osteopenia and osteoporosis are also frequent among patients on androgen deprivation therapy (ADT), which also contributes to the incidence of fractures. In this chapter, we focus on adjunct therapies for bone health for patients with prostate cancer.

ADJUNCT THERAPY FOR ADT-RELATED BONE DEMINERALIZATION

ADT increases the risk of osteopenia and osteoporosis and the risk of fractures (1). Patients may also have other risk factors such as smoking, alcohol abuse, caffeine consumption, low vitamin D level, and corticosteroid use. Usual recommendations for prevention and management include:
- Calcium/Vitamin D intake of 1,000 to 1,200 mg/800 to 1,000 IU daily. Vitamin D levels can also be measured and replaced if low.
- Weight-bearing exercise.
- Smoking cessation and limit alcohol consumption.
- Osteoclast inhibition: The timing to initiate osteoclast inhibition is unclear, but most follow the recommendations for the timing of therapy initiation and dosing similar to the management of osteoporosis. Besides bisphosphonates, denosumab can also be used in this setting (see Table 10.1) (1,2).

Table 10.1 Treatment Options for ADT-Related Osteoporosis

Zoledronic acid 5 mg intravenously every 12 mo.
Denosumab 60 mg subcutaneously every 6 mo.
Alendronate 70 mg orally weekly
Risedronate 35 mg orally weekly or 150 mg orally monthly
Ibandronate 150 mg orally monthly
Raloxifene 60 mg orally daily
ADT, androgen deprivation therapy.

- History of hip or vertebral fracture.
- T-score ≤2.5 at the femoral neck or spine by dual energy x-ray absorptiometry.
- T-score between −1 and −2.5 at the femoral neck or spine and a 10-year probability of hip fracture ≥3% or 10-year probability of any major osteoporosis-related fracture of ≥20%.

ADJUNCT THERAPY FOR PREVENTION OF BONE METASTASES

Although bisphosphonates have not been shown to prevent bone metastases, denosumab might. A phase 3 trial of 1,432 with castration resistant prostate cancer that were nonmetastatic were randomized to denosumab 120 mg every 4 weeks or placebo (3). Patients were considered high risk for bone metastases by prostate-specific antigen (PSA) ≥8 mcg/L and/or doubling time of 10 months or less. Denosumab showed a benefit in bone-metastasis-free survival of 29.5 versus 25.2 months compared to placebo. Overall survival was similar. Osteonecrosis of the jaw occurred in 5% of patients on denosumab.

ADJUNCT THERAPY FOR MANAGEMENT OF BONE METASTASES

Osteoclast inhibition has been shown to be beneficial in the castration-resistant setting in patients with bone metastases by decreasing the rate of skeletal-related events, which is a composite of pathologic fractures, radiation therapy to the bone, surgery, and spinal cord compression. This benefit has not been replicated in the castration-sensitive setting. The following are alternatives for osteoclast inhibition:

Bisphosphonates: In a trial with 643 men with castration-resistant prostate cancer, patients were randomized to zoledronic acid 4 mg, zoledronic acid 8 mg, or placebo every 3 weeks (4). The 8 mg arm was reduced to 4 mg due to risk of renal toxicity. The median time to skeletal-related event in the zoledronic acid arm was 488 versus 321 days for placebo. At 24 months, zoledronic acid had a rate of skeletal-related events of 38% versus 49%. The zoledronic acid arm also had lower pain and analgesic scores compared to placebo. This benefit has not been replicated with other bisphosphonates like pamidronate, ibandronate, or clodronate. The main side effects of zoledronic acid include acute reactions that may last up to 14 days (arthralgias, flu-like symptoms, myalgia, and hypotension), renal insufficiency, hypocalcemia and osteonecrosis of the jaw. Although the standard therapy has been 4 mg every 4 weeks (with renal adjustment as indicated), more recent trials have looked at other dosing schedules, and every 12 weeks seems noninferior (5).

Denosumab: This is a fully humanized monoclonal antibody against the nuclear factor-kappa (RANK) ligand, which is secreted by osteoblasts to activate osteoclast precursors and bone resorption. It has been compared to zoledronic acid in a randomized double-blind phase 3 trial with 1,901 men with castration-resistant prostate cancer and bone metastases (6). Patients were assigned to denosumab 120 mg or zoledronic acid 4 mg every 4 weeks and were advised to take calcium and vitamin D supplementation. Denosumab showed a benefit in the time to first skeletal-related event of 20.7 versus 17.1 months. The rates of pathologic fracture, spinal cord compression, and need for radiation were similar. The incidence of osteonecrosis of the jaw was 2.3% in the denosumab arm and 1.3% in the zoledronic acid arm. Hypocalcemia was seen in 13% of cases with denosumab and hypophosphatemia in 25%.

> **KEY POINTS**
>
> - Patients on ADT should be risk-stratified for osteoporosis-related fractures and managed accordingly with lifestyle modifications and osteoclast inhibition if indicated.
> - Denosumab has shown some activity in delaying development of bone metastases in high-risk patients.
> - Osteoclast inhibition to prevent skeletal-related events seems to be beneficial in patients with castration resistant prostate cancer with bone metastasis. Denosumab may be slightly more effective than zoledronic acid.

REFERENCES

1. Nguyen PL, Alibhai SM, Basaria S, et al. Adverse events of androgen deprivation therapy and strategies to mitigate them. *Eur Urol.* 2015;67(5):825-836.
2. Watts NB, Adler RA, Bilezikian JP, et al. Osteoporosis in men: an Endocrine Society clinical practice guideline. *J Clin Endocrinol Metab.* 2012;97(6):1802-1822.
3. Smith MR, Saad F, Coleman R, et al. Denosumab and bone-metastasis-free survival in men with castration-resistant prostate cancer: results of a phase 3, randomised placebo-controlled trial. *Lancet.* 2012;379(9810):39-46.
4. Saad F, Gleason D, Murray R, et al. A randomized, placebo-controlled trial of zoledronic acid in patients with hormone-refractory metastatic prostate carcinoma. *JNCI.* 2002;94(19):1458-1468.
5. Himelstein AL, Qin R, Novotny PJ, et al. CALGB 90604 (Alliance): a randomized phase III study of standard dosing vs. longer interval dosing of zoledronic acid in metastatic cancer [abstract]. *J Clin Oncol.* 2015;33(Suppl), Abstract 9501.
6. Fizazi K, Carducci M, Smith M, et al. Denosumab versus zoledronic acid for treatment of bone metastases in men with castration-resistant prostate cancer: a randomised, double-blind study. *Lancet.* 2011;377(9768):813-822.

Advanced Stage Prostate Cancer: Controversies in Management

11

Jesus H. Hermosillo-Rodriguez and Nicholas Mitsiades

INTRODUCTION

In this chapter, we go into more detail's about the following controversies in management of metastatic prostate cancer:
- Timing of initiation of systemic therapy for patients with elevated prostate-specific antigen (PSA) as only evidence of disease when local therapies are no longer available.
- Timing of initiation of therapy for patients with asymptomatic low-volume metastases.
- The role of first-generation antiandrogens in castration-sensitive disease.

TIMING OF INITIATION OF THERAPY FOR PATIENTS WITH ELEVATED PSA AS ONLY EVIDENCE OF DISEASE

Case 1: A 74-year-old male was found to have Gleason's 10 prostate cancer after evaluation for elevated PSA detected in screening. He underwent prostatectomy with evidence of extraprostatic extension and negative margins. He underwent adjuvant radiation and proceeded with surveillance. PSA went from less than 0.06 ng/mL to 5.1 ng/mL. Should you recommend androgen ablation therapy?

Patients with prostate cancer who have persistently elevated PSA despite surgical treatment or radiation are considered to have persistent disease. If salvage therapy is not an option, the next question is whether the patient should receive systemic therapy with androgen deprivation therapy (ADT).

While earlier initiation might prevent prostate cancer-related morbidity and improve survival, in some cases disease can be very indolent and ADT has potential adverse effects as well. Unfortunately, there are no randomized trials concluded that have addressed this question.

In a natural history study of 201 patients on ADT with PSA progression and no radiographic evidence of metastases, median bone-metastasis-free survival was 30 months. Thirty-three percent of patients developed bone metastases at 2 years. Predictors of shorter time to bone metastasis and overall survival (OS) were baseline PSA greater than 10 ng/mL and PSA doubling time of 10 months (1). If clinical trial is not an option, these factors may be useful in making the decision about starting ADT in patients with PSA-only relapse even in the ADT-naive setting. The Cancer of the Prostate Strategic Urologic Research Endeavor (CaPSURE) database in 2012 described a series of 2,022 patients with PSA only relapse who had not been treated with ADT. 34.8% of patients had a Gleason score ≥7. After adjusting for poor prognostic factors (Gleason score, PSA velocity), there was no significant difference in OS or prostate cancer specific mortality between patients who started within 3 months of diagnosis or patients who started 2 or more years later or when they presented with metastasis, symptoms, or short PSA doubling time (defined as 6 months or less for PSA <10 ng/mL) (2). Mean time to progression was 35.8 months.

If ADT is started for these patients, there is also the consideration about whether to administer it continuously or intermittently, which is addressed further in the "Intermittent Androgen Ablation in Metastatic Prostate Cancer" subchapter.

TIMING OF INITIATION OF THERAPY FOR PATIENTS WITH ASYMPTOMATIC LOW-VOLUME METASTASES AND USE OF FIRST-GENERATION ANTIANDROGENS IN CASTRATION SENSITIVE METASTATIC PROSTATE CANCER

Case 2: A 63-year-old male was found to have a PSA of 48 ng/mL after screening evaluation. A CT scan showed evidence of right pelvic bone metastasis, with uptake on a nuclear bone scan. Biopsy of a bone lesion was consistent with prostate cancer. The patient is otherwise asymptomatic.

Question 1: Should you recommend ADT?

The study of this issue has been limited by heterogeneity in the populations included in clinical trials, different triggers on initiation of ADT, and the fact that some patients do not defer therapy as originally planned (3). Also, many of the trials did not take into account prognostic factors (Gleason score, PSA response, PSA doubling time, life expectancy) into the decision-making progress. Also, while survival is a desired outcome, other factors like disease morbidity have not been consistently examined. With these limitations known, a meta-analysis looking at this question has concluded that early ADT was associated with a decrease in prostate cancer-related death, without a benefit in OS. More clinical trials are needed to answer this question; however, the information suggests that initiation of therapy should be individualized for each patient.

Question 2: Would you recommend a first-generation antiandrogen monotherapy or combined androgen blockade to this patient?

First-generation antiandrogens (e.g., bicalutamide, flutamide, nilutamide) are competitive inhibitors of androgens. They are typically recommended as initial bridging with a gonadotropin releasing hormone (GnRH) agonist and/or after disease progression to medical or surgical castration (castration-resistant disease) (3). A meta-analysis looking at the question of using castration or antiandrogen therapy alone as initial therapy for castration-sensitive prostate cancer found a trend toward shorter OS with antiandrogen monotherapy, although it was not statistically significant (hazard ratio [HR] 1.22, 95% confidence interval [CI] 0.99–1.40) (4). Although some studies have shown a progression free survival benefit of castration combined with antiandrogens as initial therapy (combined androgen blockade), it risks higher toxicity, and the benefit has not been consistently reproduced in clinical trials. Because of this, combined androgen blockade is not widely used (5).

KEY POINTS

- For patients with PSA-only disease who are not candidates for salvage therapy, deferred ADT seems to be a reasonable option, particularly for patients with low baseline PSA (<10 ng/mL) and low doubling time (<10 months).
- For patients with asymptomatic metastatic prostate cancer with low-volume disease, there is some suggestion of prostate-cancer-related mortality benefit of early ADT.
- First-generation antiandrogen monotherapy or combined androgen blockade should not be routinely used for patients with castration-sensitive prostate cancer.

REFERENCES

1. Smith MR, Kabbinavar F, Saad F, et al. Natural history of rising serum prostate-specific antigen in men with castrate nonmetastatic prostate cancer. *J Clin Oncol.* 2005;23(13):2918-2925.
2. Garcia-Albeniz X, Chan JM, Paciorek AT, et al. Immediate versus deferred initiation of androgen deprivation therapy in prostate cancer patients with PSA-only relapse. An observational follow up study. *Eur J Cancer.* 2015;51(7):817-824.
3. Loblaw A, Virgo K, Nam R, et al. Initial hormonal management of androgen-sensitive metastatic, recurrent or progressive prostate cancer: 2007 Update of an American Society of Clinical Oncology Practice Guideline. *J Clin Oncol.* 2007;25:1596-1605.
4. Park JC, Eisenberger MA. Advances in the treatment of metastatic prostate cancer. *Mayo Clinic Proceedings.* 2015;90(12):1719-33.
5. Seidenfeld J, Samson DJ, Hasselblad V, et al. Single-therapy androgen suppression in men with advanced prostate cancer: a systematic review and meta-analysis. *Ann Intern Med.* 2000;132(7):566-577.

Advanced Prostate Cancer Survivorship Challenges and Issues 12

Jesus H. Hermosillo-Rodriguez and Nicholas Mitsiades

INTRODUCTION

Patients with metastatic prostate cancer can develop side effects from therapy that can impact their quality of life and potentially limit their lifespans. This chapter focuses on these issues.

METABOLIC AND CARDIOVASCULAR EFFECTS OF ANDROGEN DEPRIVATION THERAPY

Patients with prostate cancer on androgen deprivation therapy (ADT) can develop insulin resistance, diabetes mellitus, hyperlipidemia, osteoporosis, and cardiovascular disease (1). However, increased cardiac death related to ADT has been difficult to prove in randomized controlled trials. Regardless, men initiating ADT should be counseled on lifestyle modifications, including diet, exercise, smoking cessation, and weight loss. Pharmacologic therapy for these comorbidities should also be initiated if indicated and reasonable within the clinical setting.

COMMON PALLIATIVE CARE CHALLENGES IN PATIENTS WITH METASTATIC PROSTATE CANCER

- **Fatigue**: Frequently reported in patients receiving ADT. Multiple factors like the loss of lean muscle mass and increase in fat mass, chronic pain, psychological distress, and depression are potential contributors. Exercise with muscle-strengthening programs have been shown to reduce the frequency and severity of fatigue, and a combination of resistance training with aerobic training (15–20 minutes of cardiovascular exercise at 65%–80% of maximum heart rate — two to three times a week) can be recommended.

- **Pain from bone metastases**: The most common type of bone lesions are osteoblastic, causing pain and functional impairment and contributing to fatigue (2). Besides antitumor systemic therapy and bone-directed therapies that have been discussed in previous subchapters, other adjunct therapies can be used. Factors that are taken into account in the selection of therapy include performance status, life expectancies, disease state, and effect on quality of life:
  - Analgesics: Usually the frontline therapy.
    - Nonsteroidal anti-inflammatory drugs (NSAIDs).
    - Opiates.
    - Corticosteroids (3): The mechanism of action is likely related to decreased inflammation. The ideal agent, dose, and duration is unknown, but dexamethasone is commonly used due to its lower mineralocorticoid effect and long half-life, allowing once daily dosing (e.g., dexamethasone 4–8 mg PO daily).
    - Neuropathic pain agents (4): Some patients with bone pain have neuropathic pain features and these agents may be a useful adjunct therapy in this setting.
  - Surgery: Reserved typically for patients with impending or pathologic fracture. Bracing can be used for patients who are not candidates for surgery or have limited life expectancies.
  - Radiation therapy: Usually indicated for focal symptomatic bone metastases. A single dose of 8 Gy may be sufficient for pain control.
  - Nerve blocks: For special situations of focal pain, such as rib metastases.
  - Ablation: Usually considered for patients who are not candidates for surgery or reirradiation.
  - Percutaneous vertebral augmentation: May be prescribed for patients with pathologic vertebral fractures.
- **Vasomotor symptoms**: Most men on ADT will experience hot flashes. Although there are concerns that agents that are

effective in women may not be as effective in men, agents that have shown some benefit in men with ADT-related hot flashes include:
- Progestins: Results superior to venlafaxine on a randomized, double-blind trial.
  - Medroxyprogesterone 20 mg/day.
  - Cyproterone 100 mg/day.
- Venlafaxine 75 mg/day.
- Gabapentin 900 mg daily.
- Clonidine at doses of 0.1, 0.2, or 0.4 mg daily (5).

- **Sexual dysfunction**: Counseling the patient and his partner regarding the expectations of the impact of ADT in sexual function is key. Although therapies including phosphodiesterase inhibitors, vacuum erection devices, intracorporal injection therapy, or penile prosthesis are beneficial for some patients with erectile dysfunction related to ADT, the evidence is limited regarding the effectiveness of such therapies in this setting.
- **Osteoporosis**: Men on chronic androgen ablation may develop osteoporosis. Supplementation with calcium and vitamin D and monitoring with serial bone density scans can help to prevent complications.

KEY POINTS

- Patients with prostate cancer may experience many symptoms, from both the disease and its treatment.
- It is important to closely follow bone health, treating osteoporosis from androgen deprivation as well as pain from bone metastases.
- Fatigue, vasomotor symptoms, and sexual dysfunction can greatly impact the patient's quality of life.

REFERENCES

1. Ahmadi H, Daneshmand S. Androgen deprivation therapy: evidence-based management of side effects. *BJU International.* 2013;111(4):542-548.

2. Mercadante S. Malignant bone pain: pathophysiology and treatment. *Pain.* 1997;69:1-18.
3. Weinstein E, Arnold R. Fast facts and concepts #129: steroids in the treatment of bone pain. PCNow: Palliative Care Network of Wisconsin. Medical College of Wisconsin, May 4, 2013. https://www.mypcnow.org/blank-plpib. Accessed March 2, 2016.
4. Kerba M, Wu JS, Duan Q, et al. Neuropathic pain features in patients with bone metastases referred for palliative radiotherapy. *J Clin Oncol.* 2010;28(33):4892-4897.
5. Bressler LR, Murphy CM, Shevrin DH, et al. Use of clonidine to treat hot flashes secondary to leuprolide or goserelin. *Ann Pharmacother.* 1993;27(2):182-185.

Other Genitourinary Malignancies

KIDNEY CANCER

Kidney Cancer: Histologic Subtypes and Genetic Syndromes 13

Thiri Khin and Teresa Gray Hayes

Cancer of the kidney and renal pelvis represents 3.5% of all new cancer cases in the United States. There are approximately 63,000 new cases and almost 14,000 deaths from cancer of the kidney and renal pelvis each year (1). The rate of new cases of kidney cancer has steadily been on the rise, averaging 1.4% per year over the last 10 years, according to the National Cancer Institute's (NCI) Surveillance, Epidemiology, and End Results (SEER) database. Out of all primary kidney neoplasms, renal cell carcinoma (RCC) is the most common, comprising nearly 80% to 85% of cases. Transitional cell carcinoma of the renal pelvis is the second most common, comprising approximately 8%. RCC is a heterogeneous group of tumors with distinct pathology, histology, and different clinical presentations. RCC is classified based on morphology, cell of origin, and growth pattern and histochemical and molecular basics (2,3) (Table 13.1).

Table 13.1 Classification of RCC

Classification	Percentage	Cell of origin	Molecular basics
Clear cell carcinoma	75–85	Proximal tubule	Chromosome 3p–
Papillary carcinoma (chromophilic)	10–15	Proximal tubule	+7, +17, –Y
Chromophobe	5–10	Cortical collecting duct	Hypodiploid
Oncocytic	3–7	Cortical collecting duct	Undetermined
Collecting duct of Bellini	Very rare	Medullary collecting duct	Undetermined
Unclassified	5	–	Undetermined
RCC, renal cell carcinoma.			

CLEAR CELL CARCINOMA

Clear cell carcinoma is the most common histologic subtype of RCC. It arises from the proximal tubule of the kidney. Clear cell carcinomas are mostly solid and less commonly cystic. Clear cell carcinoma is specifically associated with the von Hippel–Lindau (VHL) syndrome.

PAPILLARY CARCINOMA

Papillary carcinoma also arises from the proximal tubule and can be further divided into type 1 and type 2. Papillary carcinoma tends to be bilateral and multifocal. Type 1 usually presents in early stage and type II presents in late stages III and IV.

CHROMOPHOBE CARCINOMA

Chromophobe carcinomas originate from the intercalating cells of the collecting duct and often have a hypodiploid number of chromosomes. They usually present at an earlier stage and have a good prognosis, with a low tendency to progress and metastasize (4).

ONCOCYTOMA

Oncocytomas are rare and invariably benign in nature. Oncocytes are large nucleated cells with dense eosinophilic cytoplasm. Like chromophobe carcinomas, oncocytomas usually originate from the intercalating cells of the collecting duct. They can coexist with other forms of RCC. Oncocytomas are usually single and unilateral but can be multiple and bilateral, as seen in tuberous sclerosis.

COLLECTING DUCT TUMORS

Collecting duct tumors of Bellini are rare but aggressive in nature. They usually present at a young age in an advanced stage (T3, T4) or as metastatic disease at diagnosis. Renal medullary carcinoma is one of the most aggressive collecting duct tumors.

This is more often seen in patients with sickle cell trait, and less commonly in those with homozygous sickle cell disease. They usually present with hematuria and resemble transitional carcinoma more than other RCCs.

SARCOMATOID RCC

Sarcomatoid differentiation can occur in all subtypes of RCC but is most commonly seen in clear cell and chromophobe subtypes. Sarcomatoid tumors are aggressive and usually show high nuclear grade (grade 4). Sarcomatoid carcinomas have a higher distant metastatic rate and lower overall survival compared to their nonsarcomatoid counterparts (5).

OTHER TUMORS OF THE KIDNEY

Other rare tumors include unclassified RCCs, lymphomas, translocation carcinomas, and mucinous tubular and spindle cell carcinomas. The latter is a very rare indolent epithelial neoplasm with tightly tubular cells with extracellular mucin and spindle cells. Primary renal cell sarcomas are extremely rare and can present as various subtypes including spindle sarcoma, leiomyosarcoma, and angioliposarcoma and are aggressive in nature (Figure 13.1).

KIDNEY CANCER AND GENETIC AND FAMILIAL PREDISPOSITION

In 1979, Cohen et al. reported a family with 10 members diagnosed with kidney cancers who had a translocation between chromosomes 3 and 8 (t3;8) (6). Recognition of the familial pattern and advances in molecular genomics have led to the discovery of various hereditary cancer syndromes associated with RCC, with 12 genes currently implicated in such syndromes. Identification of key genes in the pathogenesis of hereditary kidney cancer syndrome has allowed insight into the development of sporadic cancers and serves as a framework for developing new targeted therapy. The following are the common hereditary kidney cancer syndromes (7).

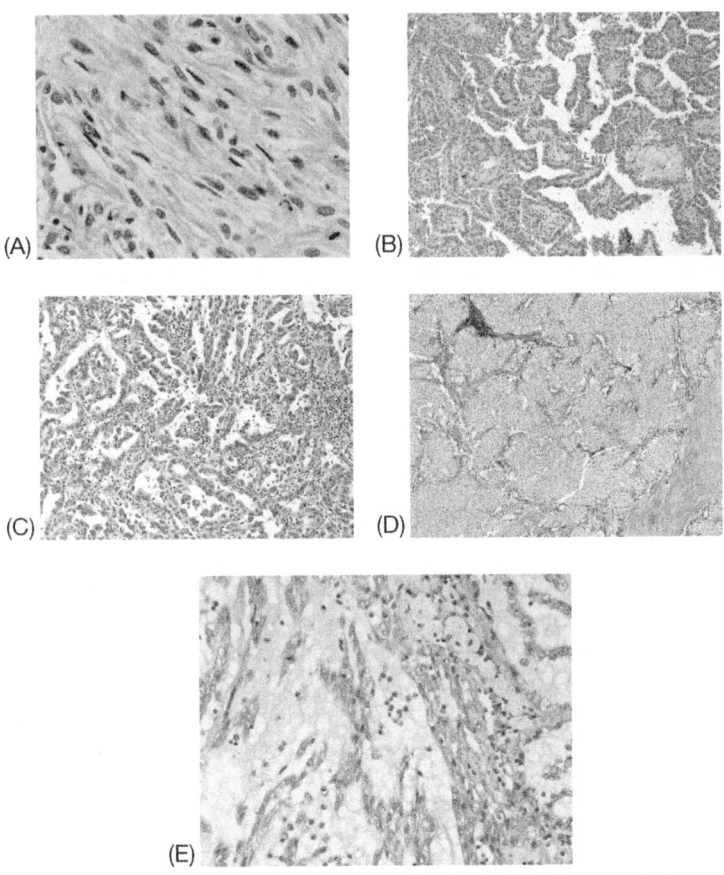

Figure 13.1 Some histologic subtypes of kidney cancer. (A) Clear cell carcinoma with sarcomatoid differentiation. (B) Papillary renal cell carcinoma. (C) Collecting duct carcinoma. (D) Chromophobe carcinoma. (E) Mucinous tubular and spindle cell carcinoma.

Source: Courtesy of Dr. Thomas Wheeler.

VON HIPPEL–LINDAU SYNDROME

VHL is an inherited, autosomal dominant syndrome caused by a germline mutation in the VHL gene, a tumor suppressor gene located in chromosome 3p. The two hit hypothesis plays a role in pathogenesis. Inheritance of an ineffective VHL allele from a parent or a de novo mutation of one allele and further deactivation of second allele lead to cyst formation and tumorigenesis.

VHL mutations are associated with a wide range of tumors, including hemangioblastomas of the brain (mainly cerebellum and spine), which is the most common type of tumor, retinal angioma, clear cell variant of RCC, pheochromocytoma, endolymphatic tumors of the middle ear, serous cystadenoma, neuroendocrine tumors of the pancreas, and papillary cystadenoma of the epididymis and broad ligament.

The VHL syndrome can be further divided into type 1 and type 2 depending on mutations and the tendency to develop certain tumors. Type 1 patients have a lower risk of pheochromocytoma. Type 2 patients have a higher risk of pheochromocytoma and can be further subclassified into type 2A with high risk of RCC, type 2B with low risk of RCC, and type 2C with only pheochromocytomas without RCC or hemangiomas.

RCC associated with VHL is invariably of the clear cell subtype and tends to be bilateral and multifocal. It usually presents before age 60. VHL gene mutation is also seen in sporadic cases of RCC. VHL gene inactivation leads to upregulation of hypoxia-inducible factors (HIF), which in turn regulates downstream vascular endothelial growth factor (VEGF) that promotes angiogenesis and proliferation. Understanding the VHL gene mutations has opened doors toward targeted treatment of VEGF in the treatment of RCC.

The management of VHL is focused on early diagnosis and appropriate intervention via thorough history taking, familial genetic screening, routine imaging, and timely surgical removal of tumor. RCC less than 3 cm in size have a low rate of metastasis and can be monitored with close surveillance. Tumors more than 3 cm require immediate surgical intervention. Nephron sparing surgery is recommended whenever possible, since tumors are often bilateral. There are ongoing trials of VEGF inhibitors in VHL patients.

HEREDITARY PAPILLARY RENAL CELL CARCINOMA

Hereditary papillary renal cell carcinoma (HPRCC) is a rare autosomal dominant familial cancer syndrome associated with the development of type I papillary renal carcinomas.

Lesions are bilateral and multifocal like other hereditary RCCs. HPRCC is caused by the HPRC gene, MET proto-oncogene, also known as hepatocyte growth factor receptor, which is located on the long arm of chromosome 7. MET gene mutation is also seen in 10% of sporadic papillary renal carcinomas.

HEREDITARY LEIOMYOMATOSIS AND RENAL CELL CARCINOMA

Hereditary leiomyomatosis and renal cell carcinoma (HLRCC) is an autosomal dominant familial cancer syndrome characterized by development of leiomyomas of the uterus and skin, and RCC. Type II papillary carcinoma is the most common tumor associated with HLRCC, but tumors of collecting ducts and chromophobe carcinomas are also seen. RCCs occur at an early age and are usually bilateral and aggressive in nature. Tumors have a high propensity to metastasize, even when as small as 1 cm in size. Uterine leiomyomas can be severe and present in up to 90% of women with HLRCC before the age of 30. Cutaneous leiomyomas are benign painful pinkish nodules of the skin, which can be disseminated throughout the body. A mutation in the fumarate hydratase gene (FH gene), which converts fumarate to malate in the Krebs cycle, is responsible for HLRCC.

BIRT–HOGG–DUBÉ SYNDROME

Birt–Hogg–Dubé syndrome (BHD) is an autosomal dominant disorder characterized by benign skin hamartomas, lung cysts and spontaneous pneumothorax, and RCC. BHD syndrome is caused by germline mutations in the folliculin gene (FLCN) located on chromosome 17p11.2, which encodes the protein folliculin. As many as 149 mutations of the FLCN gene have been identified in BHD syndrome. Skin manifestations are the earliest and most frequent manifestation of BHD syndrome. Renal cancer can occur around age 50 and is associated with different histologic subtypes, most commonly chromophobe carcinoma. Renal oncocytosis has been reported in BHD. There is also an association between BHD syndrome and colon polyposis and colorectal carcinoma.

POLYCYSTIC KIDNEY DISEASE

Polycystic kidney disease (PCKD) is a very common autosomal dominant disorder, occurring in approximately one in every 400 to 1,000 live births. RCCs in PCKD are often bilateral and multifocal, and one third are sarcomatoid type. The risk of RCC in PCKD is found to be equal to that of the general population.

TUBEROUS SCLEROSIS COMPLEX

Tuberous sclerosis complex (TSC) is an autosomal dominant disorder characterized by the formation of hamartomas in multiple organs including brain, kidney, lung, and skin. TSC is caused by mutations in one of the tumor-suppressor gene products, hamartin (TSC1) or tuberin (TSC2). The clinical manifestations include bilateral, multifocal renal lesions, which typically are angiomyolipomas. Less than 5% of patients with TSC develop RCC. This occurs at a younger age than sporadic tumors, with a female predilection. The most common histologic subtype seen in TSC is clear cell carcinoma.

PTEN HAMARTOMA TUMOR SYNDROME (COWDEN DISEASE)

Cowden disease is a rare autosomal dominant disorder causing formation of hamartomas in skin and various organs. It is associated with increased risk of tumors of breast, endometrium, and thyroid caused by mutation in the phosphatase and tensin homolog (PTEN) gene. Clear cell RCCs have been reported in patients with Cowden disease, and they usually present at a late stage.

OTHER FAMILIAL CANCER SYNDROMES WITH INCREASED RISK OF RCC

Succinate dehydrogenase (SDH) gene associated familial cancer syndrome is one of the Krebs cycle enzyme disorders. It has been reported to increase the risk of RCC in addition to hereditary paraganglioma and pheochromocytoma. Various histologic subtypes of RCC are implicated and they are usually aggressive in nature.

BAP1 (BRCA-associated protein 1) mutation in the germline predisposes to familial renal cancer and uveal and cutaneous melanomas. BAP1 is associated with a higher tumor grade and worse overall survival. Clear cell RCCs are most commonly seen.

Chromosome 3 translocation has been identified in a familial RCC as Cohen et al. reported in 1979. Multiple genes including VHL and BAP1 are located on chromosome 3p, and thus translocation and loss of alleles predispose to increased risk of RCC.

KEY POINTS

- Kidney cancers are a heterogeneous group of tumors with distinct morphology, histology, clinical presentation, and genetic predisposition.
- Knowledge of histologic subtypes and molecular basis of hereditary kidney cancer syndromes has enabled advances in the treatment of RCC patients.
- Hereditary kidney cancer syndromes account for approximately 5% of all kidney cancer cases and are mostly underdiagnosed.
- Understanding the manifestation of each subtype and its molecular pathway will assist physicians in early diagnosis and timely institution of treatment and screening for at-risk populations.

REFERENCES

1. Siegel RL, Miller KD, Jemal A. Cancer statistics, 2016. *CA Cancer J Clin.* 2016;66(1):7-30.
2. Störkel S, van den Berg E. Morphological classification of renal cancer. *World J Urol.* 1995;13(3):153-158.
3. Patard JJ, Leray E, Rioux-Leclercq N, et al. Prognostic value of histologic subtypes in renal cell carcinoma: a multicenter experience. *J Clin Oncol.* 2005;23(12):2763-2771.

4. Volpe A, Novara G, Antonelli A, et al. Chromophobe renal cell carcinoma (RCC): oncological outcomes and prognostic factors in a large multicentre series. *BJU Int.* 2012;110(1):76-83.
5. Cheville JC, Lohse CM, Kincke H, et al. Sarcomatoid renal cell carcinoma: an examination of underlying histologic subtype and an analysis of associations with patient outcome. *Am J Surg Pathol.* 2004;28(4):435-441.
6. Cohen AJ, Li FP, Berg S, et al. Hereditary renal-cell carcinoma associated with a chromosomal translocation. *N Engl J Med.* 1979;301(11):592-595.
7. Ho TH, Jonasch E. Genetic kidney cancer syndromes. *J Natl Compr Canc Netw.* 2014;12(9):1347-1355.

Treatment of Early Stage Renal Cell Carcinoma: Surgical Approaches, Partial Nephrectomy, and Ablation

14

Friedrich-Carl von Rundstedt, Wesley A. Mayer, and Richard E. Link

INTRODUCTION

For this review, "early stage disease" of renal cell carcinoma (RCC) refers to renal masses ≤7 cm (cT1, stage I) in the absence of metastasis or lymph node involvement by imaging assessment. More than 60% of small renal masses (SRM) (≤4 cm; cT1a) are incidentally detected, with imaging performed in asymptomatic patients for unrelated abdominal or musculoskeletal complaints. With the increased imaging detection of SRM there has been an overall clinical stage migration towards cT1 renal tumors. There is a direct correlation between mass size and the risk of malignancy. Smaller lesions have a higher likelihood to be benign, while larger lesions tend to be conventional clear cell carcinomas rather than the less common renal cell subtypes (papillary, chromophobe), with every centimeter in size making it more likely to be clear cell RCC.

INITIAL ASSESSMENT OF A SMALL RENAL MASS

The initial assessment of a SRM depends critically on a high quality radiographic examination. While ultrasound may provide initial suspicion for a solid renal mass, more sophisticated multiphase CT and multi parametric MRI enable one to characterize a renal mass accurately in more than 90% of all cases (Figure 14.1).

The most important criteria in the evaluation of a solid renal mass is contrast enhancement. A lesion is generally felt to be enhancing with an increase of 10 to 20 HU on the enhanced phase (arterial and venous phase) compared to

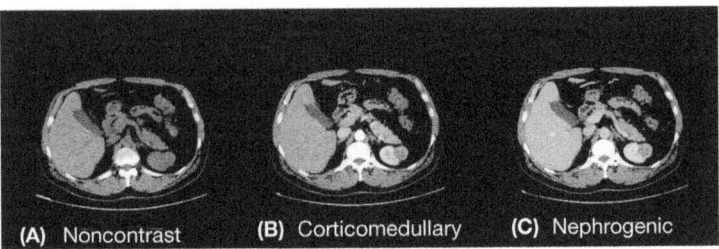
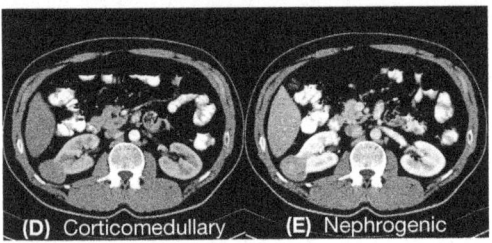

Figure 14.1 (A) Multiphasic CT allows for differentiation of renal masses. A clear cell renal carcinoma typically shows (B) strong early enhancement and (C) a washout pattern, (D and E) papillary RCC commonly demonstrates a more gradual enhancement over time.

Source: Images courtesy of Tobias Franiel MD, Department of Radiology, University Hospital Jena.

the unenhanced phase. High resolution images should provide sufficient information to plan further treatment and describe location, laterality, relationship to adjacent structures, renovascular anatomy, characteristic features, multifocality, and presence of locoregional or visceral metastasis.

SURGICAL TREATMENT

Extirpative surgical options include radical nephrectomy (RN) and partial nephrectomy (PN). Open, laparoscopic, and robotic approaches have been described for each operation.

Partial Nephrectomy

PN should be considered for all T1a and many T1b renal masses if the patient is medically fit, willing to undergo surgery, and a nephron-sparing approach is technically feasible.

There are two concepts that support the utilization of PN over RN. The first is preservation of functional nephrons. The second is mitigating the small risk of a contralateral renal tumor later in life. The risk of a contralateral tumor after a primary RCC is estimated at about 2% to 4% and will be considerably higher in patients with Von-Hippel-Lindau Disease and other familial RCC syndromes.

The primary goal of a PN is oncologic control while maximally preserving kidney function. The European Organisation for Research and Treatment of Cancer (EORTC) trial 30904 reported a lower incidence of moderate kidney disease in patients treated with a PN versus a RN but did not observe an effect on decreasing the incidence of severe chronic kidney disease (CKD) or kidney failure between the two groups (1). There was no benefit on mortality. This may be attributed to the limited median follow-up of 9.3 years. Other reports indicate an association with CKD and a higher risk of cardiovascular disease and death. While RN appears to be associated with a higher risk of CKD, it is important to recognize that progression of worsening CKD after surgical removal of nephrons may not follow the pattern of progressive decline observed in medical CKD. There is a particularly compelling rationale for nephron sparing surgery in patients with bilateral renal masses, preexisting decreased kidney function, and risk factors for progression to CKD such as diabetes and hypertension.

Note that the Guideline on SRM from the American Urology Association now recommends PN for most clinical T1 renal masses and considers oncological outcome to be "virtually identical" (2). Open, laparoscopic, and robot-assisted approaches are utilized for PN. Numerous studies failed to demonstrate a difference in oncological outcomes among the various techniques. The surgical approach, at this point, remains the surgeon's preference.

ABLATIVE TECHNIQUES

The most common ablative techniques for RCC include radiofrequency ablation (RFA) and cryotherapy, which are both thermal modalities. Ablation of a renal mass may be considered in patients with cT1a lesions. In tumors larger than 3 cm there is an increased risk of complications and local recurrence (3).

Ablation can be offered to patients not eligible for or unwilling to undergo extirpative surgery but who need or wish to receive some form of treatment. These would include very elderly or medically ill patients with rapidly growing renal masses unsuited for active surveillance. Potential advantages over extirpative surgery include decreased morbidity and shorter convalescence time. Extirpation and ablation have been reported to have similar effects on posttreatment kidney function, especially in higher risk patients with a solitary kidney (4). All ablative procedures should be preceded by a percutaneous biopsy for histological confirmation and to guide postprocedure surveillance.

Factors that guide a physician when considering an ablative approach are size, shape, and location of the lesion. In general, tumors suitable for ablation should not exceed a size of 4 cm. Proximity to critical organs such as the colon, spleen, and liver may determine feasibility of ablation. Upper pole lesions predispose to possible pleural injury. All these anatomical relationships need to be accounted for and may vary depending on the patient's position during the procedure.

For cryoablation, oncological outcomes remain controversial as there are fewer clinical trials comparing ablative procedures to extirpative approaches. Cryoablation appears to have a higher risk of recurrence as compared to PN (5). For RFA the cancer-specific survival seems to be comparable to PN in well-selected candidates (6). The challenge of all ablative techniques is the intensity of posttreatment surveillance with cross-sectional imaging. Initially, it is important to establish whether the lesion was adequately destroyed in its entirety. Most incomplete treatments (~70%) are detected within the first 3 months after ablation. As compared to PN, assessing the status of the ablated tumor may be more difficult as the lesion has not been removed but may have been rendered nonviable. Contrast enhancement of the ablated tumor is critical to determine recurrence or persistence of disease. Enhancement of the rim is less concerning than central enhancement within the tumor. The imaging characteristics of RF and cryoablated tumors may differ postprocedure.

ACTIVE SURVEILLANCE

Active surveillance (AS) of small renal tumors is an emerging concept, as about 20% of T1 enhancing renal masses are benign. Additionally, high-grade lesions are only observed in 20% to 25% of all RCCs in this size range. Many renal masses are slow growing, with an annual increase in tumor diameter of around 0.3 cm (7). There is controversy about the requirement of a renal mass biopsy prior to entering a patient into an active surveillance protocol. Some experts feel that a biopsy can be omitted for frail patients on AS where knowledge of pathology may not change management.

According to the American Urological Association Guideline (AUA), European Association of Urology (EAU), and National Comprehensive Cancer Network (NCCN) guidelines, active surveillance is primarily an option for patients unfit or unwilling to undergo surgery. This is more suitable for elderly patients with medical comorbidities and might not be a suitable option for younger, healthier patients who may prefer definitive treatment. This is reflected by the results of the Delayed Intervention and Surveillance for Small Renal Masses (DISSRM) study that prospectively enrolled 497 patients who chose active surveillance or primary active intervention. Patients on active surveillance were older, had more comorbidities, higher Eastern Cooperative Oncology Group (ECOG) scores, smaller tumors, and more often multiple or bilateral lesions. Cancer-specific survival was 99% and 100% respectively in this cohort, supporting active surveillance as an oncologically viable and safe option for well-selected patients (8). There are no universally accepted criteria to determine who is a candidate for AS. Wolf et al. proposed a biopsy-directed management algorithm that utilizes histology and grading to designate patients for surveillance or intervention. While this is a very pragmatic approach, it has not yet been validated in a randomized clinical trial (9).

RENAL MASS BIOPSY

Histological confirmation of RCC is not a requirement during the diagnostic work-up of a solid enhancing renal mass. Currently, imaging more than histological diagnosis generally determines the choice of a definitive management. A renal biopsy should be performed as a core needle biopsy, which has a higher sensitivity and specificity than fine needle aspiration (10). Renal biopsy performs poorly for cystic lesions and for tumors smaller than 1 cm. The biopsy can be performed using ultrasound, CT, or MRI guidance. A renal mass biopsy has a complication rate of up to 8%. Complications are mostly related to bleeding, pain, infection, or injury of adjacent structures. Tumor seeding is an extremely rarely reported event, with only three reported cases in the last 25 years.

The true risk of a renal mass biopsy is a false negative result. Biopsies may also either miss the lesion or not collect enough viable tissue for a histopathological diagnosis. Also, it is critical to recognize that renal tumors show tremendous intratumoral heterogeneity, so a single biopsy may not adequately reflect the true malignant potential of a given tumor. The previously referenced meta-analysis reported sensitivity and specificity of 99.1% and 99.7%, respectively. A correct histological diagnosis is achieved in about 83% of cases.

The management of SRM requires an interdisciplinary treatment approach. Open and comprehensive communication among the radiologist, pathologist, urologist, medical oncologist, and interventional radiologist will improve patient selection and individual outcomes.

KEY POINTS

- More than 60% of all SRM are incidentally detected. About 20% of all lesions have a benign histology.
- Contrast enhanced CT or MRI are the preferred imaging modalities for localized RCC.
- PN is the preferred surgical option for all pT1a lesions and should be considered for pT1b lesions.
- Active surveillance or ablative treatments with cryotherapy or RFA are management options for elderly or frail patients, or patients with comorbidities.
- Renal biopsy is recommended prior to ablative therapies and may be considered for active surveillance strategies

REFERENCES

1. Scosyrev E, Messing EM, Sylvester R, et al. Renal function after nephron-sparing surgery versus radical nephrectomy: results from EORTC randomized trial 30904. *Eur Urol.* 2014;65:372-377.
2. Novick AC, Campbell SC, Belldegrun A, et al. AUA Guideline for Management of the Clinical Stage 1 Renal Mass. https://www.auanet.org/education/guidelines/renal-mass.cfm. Accessed October 10, 2016.
3. Best S., Park SK, Youssef RF, et al. Long-term outcomes of renal tumor radio frequency ablation stratified by tumor diameter: size matters. *J Urol.* 2012;187:1183-1189.
4. Mues AC, Korets R., Graversen JA, et al. Clinical, pathologic, and functional outcomes after nephron-sparing surgery in patients with a solitary kidney: a multicenter experience. *J Endourol.* 2012;26:1361-1366.
5. Rodriguez Faba O, Akdogan B, Marszalek M, et al. Current status of focal cryoablation for small renal masses. *Urology.* 2016;90:9-15.
6. Chang X., Zhang F, Liu T, et al. Radio frequency ablation versus partial nephrectomy for clinical T1b renal cell carcinoma: long-term clinical and oncologic outcomes. *J Urol.* 2015;193(2):430-435.
7. Smaldone MC, Kutikov A, Egleston BL, et al. Small renal masses progressing to metastases under active surveillance: a systematic review and pooled analysis. *Cancer.* 2012;118:997-1006.
8. Pierorazio PM, Johnson MH, Ball MW, et al. Five-year analysis of a multi-institutional prospective clinical trial of delayed intervention and surveillance for small renal masses: the DISSRM registry. *Eur Urol.* 2015;68:408-415.
9. Halverson SJ, Kunju LP, Bhalla R, et al. Accuracy of determining small renal mass management with risk stratified biopsies: confirmation by final pathology. *J Urol.* 2013;189:441-446.
10. Marconi L, Dabestani S, Lam TB, et al. Systematic review and meta-analysis of diagnostic accuracy of percutaneous renal tumour biopsy. *Eur Urol.* 2016;69:660-673.

Renal Cell Carcinoma: Treatment of Advanced Kidney Cancer   15

Kanza S. Abbas and Teresa Gray Hayes

INTRODUCTION

Surgical resection is a good curative option for localized renal cell carcinoma (RCC), but the cancer often recurs or presents as metastatic cancer due to the silent nature of the disease. Once metastatic, the disease is generally not curable, but there are many palliative options. Therapeutic options for metastatic clear cell RCC include immunotherapy, molecularly targeted agents, surgery, and radiation.

THERAPEUTIC OPTIONS AND APPROACH

For newly diagnosed or newly metastatic RCC patients, we need to keep in mind the histology of the tumor as well as risks that stratify them. More than 60% of patients with RCC have clear cell histology. Patients are deemed poor risk if they have three or more of the following criteria (CHALKS):

C = Calcium greater than 10 (corrected calcium)

H = Hemoglobin less than normal

A = Absence of kidney (or interval of <1 year between diagnosis and systemic therapy)

L = LDH greater than 1.5 × normal

K = Karnofsky performance status (KPS) less than 80%

S = Sites of metastatic disease greater than two

IMMUNOTHERAPY

Immunotherapy is an important option for the management of patients with advanced clear cell RCC, both as initial therapy or as secondary therapy after molecularly targeted therapy. High-dose bolus IL-2 can activate an immune response against RCC that results in prolonged tumor regression in a minority of patients. Although treatment with high-dose IL-2 is associated with severe toxicity and requires specialized centers, it is also the only therapy that can provide long-term remission in certain patients, even in the absence of additional therapy. Therefore, it is an important option for carefully selected patients. Good candidates for high-dose IL-2 have excellent performance status, clear cell histology, and minimal metastatic disease burden.

Other immunotherapy options that are upcoming are PDL1 and PD1 inhibitors. Nivolumab has shown prolonged overall survival (OS) compared to everolimus as a second-line therapy and is now being employed as a second line therapy once patients fail targeted therapy. Interferon alpha (IFN-α) is another option that was previously used but has now been largely replaced by newer immunotherapy and targeted options due to partial and shorter responses.

TARGETED THERAPIES

VEGF Inhibitors: These agents work by targeting the vascular endothelial growth factor (VEGF) pathway. They are either small molecule tyrosine kinase inhibitors (TKIs) like sunitinib, pazopanib, cabozantinib, axitinib, or sorafenib, or a monoclonal antibody such as bevacizumab. TKIs prolong OS compared with IFN-α for the initial management of advanced RCC and are also active in the treatment of patients with disease progression after cytokine therapy. Therefore, they are the preferred first-line treatment in the majority of patients except when the patient is a candidate for IL-2 or when the patient's disease falls in the poor risk category. In the absence of prior immunotherapy, generally treatment is started off with sunitinib, pazopanib, or a combination of bevacizumab and IFN-α. Sunitinib and pazopanib are generally preferred and have similar efficacy (Table 15.1).

If prior immunotherapy has been used as first-line therapy, TKIs can be employed as second-line. Axitinib is the slightly preferred option as it is the most selective of the VEGF TKIs, but pazopanib or sunitinib can also be used.

Once a patient's cancer has progressed on a first-line TKI, immunotherapy (nivolumab) can be used, but other TKIs such as cabozantinib can also be employed. The previously mentioned TKIs also remain an option, as does sorafenib. While a number of agents are available, data is limited in comparing them to each other, especially in the second-line and subsequent settings (Table 15.2).

mTOR inhibitors: The mTOR pathway is downstream of the phosphoinositide 3-kinase and Akt pathway. Current mTOR inhibitors include temsirolimus and everolimus. The principal utility for temsirolimus in RCC is as first-line therapy for poor risk RCC or for those with mutations in the PI3K pathway. Everolimus may be used in patients whose disease is

Table 15.1 First-Line Treatment Options for Clear Cell RCC

Risk status	Preferred treatment options	Alternate options
Non-poor risk	Pazopanib Sunitinib IFN-α and Bevacizumab	High-dose IL-2 Axitinib
Poor risk	Temsirolimus	Sunitinib

IFN-α, interferon alpha; IL-2, interleukin-2; RCC, renal cell carcinoma.

Table 15.2 Second-Line Treatment Options for Clear Cell RCC

Prior first line therapy	Preferred second line therapy	Other options
TKI	Nivolumab (preferred) Everolimus Axitinib	Pazopanib Sorafenib Sunitinib
Immunotherapy (IL-2/IFN based)	Axitinib (Preferred) Sunitinib Pazopanib Sorafenib	Temsirolimus Bevacizumab
mTOR inhibitor		Clinical trial TKI

IFN, interferon; IL-2, interleukin-2; mTOR, mechanistic target of rapamycin; RCC, renal cell carcinoma; TKI, tyrosine kinase inhibitors.

refractory to initial treatment with VEGF receptor TKIs and/or those patients whose tumors have mutations in the PI3K pathway. However, it cannot replace temsirolimus for poor risk disease.

CHEMOTHERAPY AND HORMONAL THERAPY

Both chemotherapy and progestational agents had only very limited activity in early studies prior to the development of immunotherapy and molecularly targeted therapy, and are generally not employed in treatment of clear cell RCC currently.

SYSTEMIC THERAPY OF NON-CLEAR CELL CARCINOMA

The activity of molecularly targeted agents (sunitinib, sorafenib, and temsirolimus) in patients with non-clear cell RCC is based primarily on Phase 2 studies and meta-analysis and show that these agents have limited activity. These patients do not respond to cytokine-based immunotherapy. Some case reports exist for nivolumab in papillary RCC with sarcomatoid features, although confirmatory data are needed before such a treatment approach can be endorsed. Some of these tumors are chemosensitive. Responses have been reported with combinations of platinum agents, taxanes, gemcitabine, or ifosfamide in patients with collecting duct tumors and sarcomatoid RCCs. Renal medullary carcinoma may also be responsive to platinum-based combination chemotherapy regimens, anthracyclines, or bortezomib.

SURGERY

Most patients with stage IV RCC have unresectable disease and require systemic therapy. However, for patients in whom the only evidence of advanced disease is the direct involvement of the ipsilateral adrenal gland, a radical nephrectomy that includes adrenalectomy is potentially curative. The removal of the primary tumor (cytoreductive or debulking nephrectomy) should be performed in all patients when it is clinically feasible and justifiable (good performance status, 75% debulking possible, no symptomatic metastatic disease) before initiating systemic therapy, as this results in improved survival. Surgical resection of a single or limited number of metastases in conjunction with a radical nephrectomy may be performed in selected patients.

RADIATION THERAPY

Although RCC has been characterized as a radioresistant tumor, conventional and stereotactic radiation therapy (RT) are frequently useful to treat a single or limited number of metastases for purposes of pain control, bone metastases, or brain metastases.

KEY POINTS

- IL-2 remains a first-line option for carefully selected patients. For most others, a molecularly targeted agent like pazopanib or sunitinib is the agent of choice.
- For patients who progress on immunotherapy, axitinib or other TKIs may be used next line. For patients who progress on VEGF inhibitors, treatment with nivolumab or cabozantinib is next.
- After second-line therapy, any of the abovementioned regimens may be used including axitinib, cabozantinib, everolimus, or sorafenib. Patients should be encouraged to participate in formal clinical trials whenever possible.
- For non-clear cell RCC, targeted therapy should be employed. However, chemotherapy may be used in specific subtypes such as collecting duct, sarcomatoid, and medullary carcinoma, which may be chemosensitive.
- Radiation and cytoreductive nephrectomies can be done in selected patients depending on disease site, burden, and number of treatments received.

RECOMMENDED READING

- De Velasco G, Hamieh L, Micjkey S, Choueiri TK1. Optimizing systemic therapy for metastatic renal cell carcinoma beyond the first line setting. *Urol Oncol.* 2015;33(12):538-545.
- Escudier B, Gore M. Sequencing therapy in metastatic renal cell cancer. *Semin Oncol.* 2013;40(4):465-471.
- Motzer RJ, Escudier B, McDermott DF, et al. Nivolumab versus everolimus in advanced renal-cell carcinoma. *N Engl J Med.* 2015;373(19):1803-1813.

Controversies in the Surgical Management of Renal Cell Carcinoma 16

Thomas E. Stout and Samit D. Soni

Case 1: A 63-year-old male is diagnosed with a left renal mass 12 cm in maximal diameter, with extension into the perirenal fat. Staging imaging shows no evidence of lymphatic involvement or distant metastasis. He is scheduled to undergo a left radical nephrectomy.

Question 1: Should this patient additionally undergo a regional lymph node dissection, and if so, to what extent?
While the indications for lymph node dissection (LND) are well established in the treatment of other urologic cancers, the utility of regional LND for renal cell carcinoma (RCC) remains controversial. The incidence of isolated retroperitoneal lymph node (LN) metastases has been cited to be less than 10% (1). The European Organization for Research and Treatment of Cancer (EORTC) 30881 is the only randomized study to date that has addressed the role of regional LND in the setting of radical nephrectomy (RN) for RCC, and 732 patients with preoperative N0M0 tumors were eligible (2). With a median follow-up period of 12.6 years, regional LND did not improve cure or survival in patients that underwent RN for T1 to T3 diseases. In this cohort, regional nodal metastases were present in 1% of palpably normal nodes and 17% of palpably abnormal nodes, and LND did not increase the risk of perioperative complications.

However, certain limitations do exist in the EORTC 30881 trial. In particular, although the trial enrolled 732 patients, given the small proportion of patients with positive LN status, the study was underpowered to conclude that the outcomes were equivalent. In addition, data such as the number of regional LNs resected and the number of positive LNs were also not included or analyzed in the study.

While the EORTC study concluded that the added benefit of LND is marginal in patients without clinically abnormal LNs, several retrospective studies suggest that patients with N1 RCC may have improved cancer-specific survival (CSS) and response to adjuvant immunotherapy following LND (3). It has been shown that increasing the number of LNs removed by 10 improves CSS in patients with N1 disease by 10% at 5 years (4). Therefore, in patients with a high risk of nodal metastases, a regional LND may be warranted. Patients considered to be high risk include those with ≥2 of the following risk factors: grade 3 to 4, stage T3 to T4, tumor size ≥ 10 cm, tumor necrosis, and sarcomatoid elements (5).

The most common location of nodal involvement is the interaortocaval nodes in right-sided tumors and the para-aortic nodes in left-sided tumors. Dissection templates should extend from the diaphragmatic crus to the common iliac artery and include paracaval and interaortocaval nodes for right-sided tumors and para-aortic and interaortocaval nodes for left-sided tumors (6).

Case 2: A 71-year-old female is diagnosed with a 13.4 cm right renal mass. Staging workup reveals a 2 cm hepatic nodule and several sub-centimeter right-sided pulmonary lesions. The patient is to be treated with six cycles of bevacizumab + IFN-α.

Question 2: Would this patient benefit from a cytoreductive nephrectomy prior to systemic therapy?

The argument for cytoreductive nephrectomy (CN) was originally developed in the era of systemic immunotherapy. Based on the results of two randomized clinical trials Southwest Oncology Group (SWOG) and EORTC, patients with metastatic RCC (mRCC) with resectable primary tumors without brain metastases and who are medically fit (Eastern Cooperative Oncology Group [ECOG] 0–1) appear to demonstrate improvement in time-to-progression and overall survival when treated with CN prior to systemic interferon (IFN). SWOG 8949 demonstrated a median survival increase of 3 months (11.1 vs. 8.1 months) in 246 patients who were randomized to either IFN-α only or CN with postoperative IFN-α. These findings were independent of performance status, metastatic site, or the presence of metastatic lesions. However, a performance status of 0 was associated with a 10-month median increase in overall survival when compared to a performance status of 1 within the CN cohort (7). Meanwhile, the EORTC study showed a survival advantage of 10 months overall (17 vs. 7 months) favoring combination therapy over interferon therapy alone (8). The rate of perioperative mortality was also very low at less than 1%. Flanigan et al subsequently performed a combined analysis of these two studies and found a 6-month overall survival benefit (13.6 vs. 7.8 months) favoring combined CN and immunotherapy. In addition, Lara et al reevaluated the SWOG data with 9-year long-term follow-up data and found a consistent 3-month survival benefit, or a 26% reduction in death. On multivariate analysis, performance status (1 vs. 0), elevated alkaline phosphatase, and lung metastasis were independent predictors of overall survival (9).

Question 3: If the above patient was instead being treated with sunitinib, would she benefit from a cytoreductive nephrectomy?

In the era of targeted therapy for RCC with agents such as tyrosine kinase, mechanistic targets of rapamycin, and vascular endothelial growth factor inhibitors (mechanistic target of rapamycin [mTOR], and vascular endothelial growth factor [VEGF] inhibitors), similar prospective studies have yet to be completed. Targeted therapy has proven itself to be significantly superior to cytokine therapy, and this has resulted in some controversy as to whether concomitant CN is beneficial in patients already receiving targeted therapy. You et al retrospectively reported their results comparing outcomes for 78 patients with mRCC who underwent targeted therapy alone or who had CN as well. Although the CN group did have a median overall survival of 21.6 months compared to 13.9 months in the control group, this was not statistically significant according to the authors (10). In contrast, Choueiri et al performed a multi-institutional study that did demonstrate a statistically significant improvement in median overall survival (19.8 vs. 94 months) in mRCC patients with favorable or intermediate prognostic features who underwent CN. These features include performance score (>80), age less than 75 years, more than one site of metastatic disease, and no brain metastasis (11). Patients with poor prognostic features only realized a marginal benefit from CN, indicating that CN should only be reserved for palliative purposes in such cases.

It is critical to point out that nearly all patients enrolled in the original clinical trials that assessed efficacy of the currently available targeted agents were completed in the setting of a prior nephrectomy. Therefore, the clinical efficacy of these targeted agents has only been evaluated in the context of a resected primary tumor. The CARMENA phase 3 trial is an ongoing clinical trial that will hopefully provide the much-needed insight into the role of CN in the era of targeted therapy.

Case 3: A 68-year-old male with a solitary left kidney is found to have a 9.7 cm exophytic renal mass. Metastatic workup demonstrates a 1.5 cm left pulmonary nodule and multiple osteolytic bone lesions, and his estimated glomerular filtration rate (eGFR) is greater than 60.

Question 4: What is the role of cytoreductive nephron-sparing surgery in this patient?

The role of nephron-sparing surgery (NSS) for cytoreductive therapy in the setting of mRCC is less well studied. Several retrospective case series have reported the use of NSS in the setting of mRCC, but no high-quality studies exist. As preservation of renal function is important in the context of potentially nephrotoxic drugs used for mRCC, NSS may be a reasonable alternative to CN in patients with underlying renal dysfunction or other imperative reasons for NSS (i.e., solitary kidney or bilateral tumors).

The four largest retrospective studies evaluating the role of NSS in patients with mRCC include between 16 and 70 patients, and have yielded mixed results. The first such study retrospectively identified 16 patients from the Mayo Clinic Nephrectomy Registry, 12 of whom had a solitary kidney, who underwent NSS for pM1 RCC. CSS rates were comparable to patients who had undergone RN for pM1 disease; however, early and late complication rates were higher in the 12 solitary kidney patients (12). Capitanio et al used the Surveillance, Epidemiology, and End Results (SEER) cancer registry to identify 46 patients with mRCC who were treated with RN or NSS, respectively, and found no difference in CSS in matched and unmatched regression analyses (13). In another mRCC study comparing 45 NSS cases to 732 RN cases, RN led to a 1.7-fold and 1.5-fold higher RCC-specific mortality in unmatched and matched analyses, respectively. However, the results were not statistically significant (14). A fourth retrospective study by Hellenthal et al actually found improved CSS in patients undergoing NSS for mRCC. In this study, the authors evaluated 8,498 patients with mRCC from the SEER database, of which 2,950 underwent cytoreductive surgery. While the vast majority of patients (98%) underwent cytoreductive RN, 70 patients (with tumors 2–3 cm in size) underwent cytoreductive partial nephrectomy. Although multivariate analysis was utilized to account for preoperative risk factors, those patients undergoing NSS were found to be 0.49 times as likely to die of RCC as those who underwent RN (15).

It is important to note that several of these studies were population based and contained limited information regarding clinical and patient information. Also, due to the small sample sizes in these studies, other prognostic variables on CSS, such as performance status and LN status, were unable to be controlled. Finally, these results may at least partially be attributed to the difference in tumor burden between patients undergoing NSS and RN.

Patients with a solitary kidney and pM1 disease undergoing NSS have been shown to have an increased rate of early and late complications compared to patients undergoing RN; however, this increase may be due to underlying medical conditions such as chronic renal insufficiency that necessitated NSS in this population. In one analysis of 33 patients with mRCC, those who underwent NSS for metachronous contralateral renal masses and a renal mass ≤ 4 cm had longer overall survival compared to those with bilateral synchronous or unilateral renal masses, likely because patients presenting with synchronous renal tumors were more often metastatic at the time of presentation (16). While further research is needed, the primary tumor burden compared to the metastatic burden, and the time lag between the index tumor and subsequent masses may guide the decision to proceed with cytoreductive RN or NSS for mRCC.

Case 4: A 61-year-old female is diagnosed with a right-sided T3aN0M1 renal cell carcinoma. Percutaneous renal mass biopsy demonstrates papillary type II histology, Fuhrman grade III.

Question 5: Should this patient undergo a cytoreductive radical nephrectomy?
While nonclear cell (ncc) histology following nephrectomy for localized disease predicts a favorable prognosis, metastatic nccRCC is characterized by poor prognosis and resistance to

chemotherapy. Kassouf et al compared outcomes of 92 patients who underwent CN for metastatic nccRCC against 514 patients who underwent CN for metastatic clear cell RCC (ccRCC) (17). The 2-year overall survival rate in patients with nccRCC was 24% compared to 44% in those with clear cell histology. Nodal disease predicted a worse outcome in patients with ccRCC but was not an independent predictor in the nccRCC cohort, despite the higher incidence of node positivity in that group. Due to the paucity of nccRCC compared to clear cell histology, the relative proportion of patients with ncc histology in clinical trials is typically less than 10%. As a result, there is a lack of strong clinical data on the role of RN or NSS for metastatic disease in this subpopulation.

Case 5: A 66-year-old male with diabetes mellitus and chronic kidney disease (CKD) stage IIIB is found to have a 11.4 cm largely exophytic right renal mass with evidence of invasion into the surrounding Gerota's fat.

Question 6: Is this patient a candidate for a cytoreductive nephrectomy?

While NSS is routinely utilized in patients with primary renal masses less than 7 cm (stage T1), RN has largely remained the treatment of choice for patients with locally advanced disease (stage T2–T4). However, several studies have examined the potential role of NSS in patients with locally advanced RCC. Margulis et al reviewed 26 patients who underwent NSS for clinical T3a or T3b tumors, mostly due to imperative indications such as solitary kidney, atrophic contralateral kidney, or chronic renal insufficiency (18). When adjusted for grade, stage, size, and tumor histology, NSS did not adversely impact disease recurrence or RCC-specific death compared to RN. NSS was associated with higher procedure-related complications, but similar blood loss, transfusion rates, and hospital length of stay compared to RN. The authors did not comment on the differences between the two groups regarding the need for long-term dialysis or the ability to receive systemic therapy. Likewise, Kolla et al showed comparable recurrence-free survival rates in six of seven patients who underwent NSS for T3b disease, without the need for dialysis at a mean follow-up time of 30 months (19). In another study, Angermeier et al retrospectively reviewed nine patients who underwent NSS for tumors with venous involvement. Five patients had no evidence of disease at a median follow-up of 33 months and the remaining four died of metastatic disease at a median time of 35.5 months postoperatively (20).

As locally advanced RCC is associated with an increased risk of contralateral tumor development and systemic relapse, select patients with solitary kidneys or chronic renal insufficiency may be suitable candidates for an attempt at NSS. NSS in the setting of locally advanced disease is technically challenging and associated with longer ischemia times and increased likelihood of postoperative renal dysfunction. Thus, careful preoperative planning and intraoperative ultrasound should be stressed in these complicated cases.

Case 6: A 69-year-old female is found to have a 3 cm exophytic right upper pole and a 4 cm exophytic right interpolar renal mass. She has no history of hereditary syndromes associated with renal tumors, her metastatic workup is negative, and her eGFR is 55.

Question 7: Is this patient a candidate for NSS, and if NSS were to be performed, when would one consider converting to a radical nephrectomy?

Although there is some consensus regarding the surgical management of patients with hereditary syndromes such as Von-Hippel Lindau and familial papillary RCC, there are no clear guidelines on the surgical management of patients found to have sporadic multifocal tumors. While patients with hereditary RCC often present with multifocal disease, sporadic cases are multifocal in only 3% to 20% of patients (21,22). Multifocal cases of sporadic RCC are also usually more advanced at the time of diagnosis and have higher recurrence rates than their solitary counterparts. Nonhereditary multifocal cases are traditionally treated with RN due to these factors; however, the role of NSS has been investigated in three large retrospective studies. Two studies performed at a single institution compared outcomes of NSS and RN for sporadic, multiple, ipsilateral renal tumors. The 5-year CSS was comparable between both groups and the recurrence rates with NSS were between 10% and 13% (23,24). Mano et al. analyzed 78 patients who underwent NSS and 45 patients who underwent RN for nonmetastatic, unilateral, synchronous, multifocal renal tumors (25). Five-year recurrence-free survival rates were 98% and 85% in the NSS and RN groups, respectively. Of note, however, cases in the RN group had significantly larger primary tumor burden, higher pathologic T stages, and higher RENAL nephrometry scores. The rate of postoperative complications was comparable between the two groups and kidney function was preserved in 75% of NSS patients at 5 years. These data suggest that with careful surgical selection, NSS produces equivalent survival rates for multifocal sporadic tumors as RN. If NSS is to be performed, the surgeon should be prepared to convert to RN in the presence of extensive tumor burden, large resections resulting in inadequate residual kidney, or adverse intraoperative pathology of satellite lesions.

KEY POINTS

1. For clinical stage N1 RCC, retrospective data suggest that LND may improve CSS, but the prospective EORTC study did not demonstrate such a benefit.
2. Patients with mRCC who have a good performance status have improved survival with cytoreductive RN prior to systemic treatment with interferon. However, such clinical studies have not been performed in the era of targeted therapy, and the specific subset of patients with mRCC who may benefit from cytoreductive therapy prior to targeted therapy has yet to be established.
3. Although prospective clinical studies have not been performed to date, cytoreductive NSS may be a reasonable alternative to cytoreductive RN in patients with underlying renal dysfunction or solitary kidney.
4. The 2-year overall survival rate in patients undergoing CN for metastatic ncc RCC is 24% compared to 44% in those with clear cell histology.
5. As locally advanced RCC is associated with an increased risk of contralateral tumor development and systemic relapse, patients with solitary kidneys or underlying renal insufficiency may be suitable candidates for NSS.
6. Early data show that NSS for sporadic, multifocal renal tumors may have comparable oncologic outcomes to RN in carefully selected patients.

REFERENCES

1. Minervini A, Lilas L, Morelli G, et al. Regional lymph node dissection in the treatment of renal cell carcinoma: is it useful in patients with no suspected adenopathy before or during surgery? *BJU Int.* 2001;88(3):169-172.
2. Blom JH, van Poppel H, Marécheal JM, et al. Radical nephrectomy with and without lymph-node dissection: final results of European Organization for Research and Treatment of Cancer (EORTC) randomized phase 3 trial 30881. *Eur Urol.* 2009;55(1):28-34.
3. Pantuck AJ, Zisman A, Dorey F, et al. Renal cell carcinoma with retroperitoneal lymph nodes: role of lymph node dissection. *J Urol.* 2003;169(6):2076-2083.
4. Whitson JM, Harris CR, Reese AC, et al. Lymphadenectomy improves survival of patients with renal cell carcinoma and nodal metastases. *J Urol.* 2011;185(5):1615-1620.
5. Hutterer GC, Patard JJ, Ionescu C, et al. Patients with renal cell carcinoma nodal metastases can be accurately identified: external validation of a new nomogram. *Int J Cancer.* 2007;121(11):2556-2561.
6. Crispen PL, Breau RH, Allmer C, et al. Lymph node dissection at the time of radical nephrectomy for high-risk clear cell renal cell carcinoma: indications and recommendations for surgical templates. *J Urol.* 2011;59(1):18-23.
7. Flanigan RC, Salmon SE, Blumenstein BA, et al. Nephrectomy followed by interferon alfa-2b compared with interferon alfa-2b alone for metastatic renal-cell cancer. *N Engl J Med.* 2001;345(23):1655-1659.
8. Mickisch GH, Garin A, van Poppel H, et al. Radical nephrectomy plus interferon-alfa-based immunotherapy compared with interferon alfa alone in metastatic renal-cell carcinoma: a randomised trial. *Lancet.* 2001;358(9286):966-970.
9. Lara Jr. PN, Tangen CM, Conlon S, et al. Predictors of survival in advanced renal cell carcinoma: long-term results from southwest oncology group trial S8949. *J Urol.* 2009;181(2):512-517.
10. You D, Jeong IG, Ahn JH, et al. The value of cytoreductive nephrectomy for metastatic renal cell carcinoma in the era of targeted therapy. *J Urol.* 2011;185(1):54-59.
11. Choueiri TK, Xie W, Kollmannsberger C, et al. The impact of cytoreductive therapy on survival of patients with metastatic renal cell carcinoma receiving vascular endothelial growth factor targeted therapy. *J Urol.* 2011;185(1):60-66.
12. Krambeck AE, Leibovich BC, Lohse CM, et al. The role of nephron sparing surgery for metastatic (pM1) renal cell carcinoma. *J Urol.* 2006;176(5):1990-1995.
13. Capitanio U, Zini L, Perrotte P, et al. Cytoreductive partial nephrectomy does not undermine cancer control in metastatic renal cell carcinoma: a population-based study. *Urology.* 2008;72(5):1090-1095.

14. Hutterer GC, Patard JJ, Colombel M, et al. Cytoreductive nephron-sparing surgery does not appear to undermine disease-specific survival in patients with metastatic renal cell carcinoma. *Cancer.* 2007;110(11):2428-2433.
15. Hellenthal NJ, Mansour AM, Hayn MH, et al. Is there a role for partial nephrectomy in patients with metastatic renal cell carcinoma? *Urol Oncol.* 2013;31(1):36-41.
16. Babaian KN, Merrill MM, Matin S, et al. Partial nephrectomy in the setting of metastatic renal cell carcinoma. *J Urol.* 2014;192(1):36-42.
17. Kassouf W, Sanchez-Ortiz R, Tamboli P, et al. Cytoreductive nephrectomy for metastatic renal cell carcinoma with nonclear cell histology. *J Urol.* 2007;178(5):1896-1900.
18. Margulis V, Tamboli P, Jacobsohn KM, et al. Oncological efficacy and safety of nephron-sparing surgery for selected patients with locally advanced renal cell carcinoma. *BJU Int.* 2007;100(6):1235-1239.
19. Kolla SB, Ercole C, Spiess PE, et al. Nephron-sparing surgery for pathological stage T3b renal cell carcinoma confined to the renal vein. *BJU Int.* 2010;106(10):1494-1498.
20. Angermeier KW, Novick AC, Streem SB, et al. Nephron-sparing surgery for renal cell carcinoma with renal involvement. *J Urol.* 1990;144(6):1352-1355.
21. Richstone L, Scheer DS, Reuter VR, et al. Multifocal renal cortical tumors: frequency, associated clinicopathological features and impact on survival. *J Urol.* 2004;171(2):615-620.
22. Tsivian M, Moreira DM, Caso JR, et al. Predicting occult multifocality of renal cell carcinoma. *Eur Urol.* 2010;58(1):118-126.
23. Blute ML, Thibault GP, Leibovich BC, et al. Multiple ipsilateral renal tumors discovered at planned nephron sparing surgery: importance of tumor histology and risk of metachronous recurrence. *J Urol.* 2003;170(3):760-763.
24. Krambeck A, Iwaszko M, Leibovich B, et al. Long-term outcome of multiple ipsilateral renal tumours found at the time of planned nephron-sparing surgery. *BJU Int.* 2008;101(11):1375-1379.
25. Mano R, Kent M, Larish Y, et al. Partial and radical nephrectomy for unilateral synchronous multifocal renal cortical tumors. *J Urol.* 2015;85(6):1404-1410.

Investigational Technologies in the Surgical Management of Renal Cell Carcinoma 17

Thomas E. Stout and Samit D. Soni

HIGH INTENSITY FOCUSED ULTRASOUND

Just as there have been a multitude of advances in immunotherapy and targeted therapy for advanced renal cell carcinoma (RCC), new developments exist in the treatment of localized disease. Cryoablation and radiofrequency ablation (RFA) are well-established therapies for the treatment of small tumors less than 4 cm in patients who are considered poor surgical candidates (1). High-intensity focused ultrasound (HIFU) is another thermo-ablative technique for extracorporeal ablation of small renal masses. High-intensity ultrasound waves increase tissue temperatures to greater than 65°C and damage targeted tissue by thermal and acoustic cavitation (2). Compared to cryoablation and RFA, extracorporeal HIFU is entirely noninvasive, and the purely externally focused ablation eliminates the risk of tumor spillage or hemorrhage due to needle placement. Additionally, heat generation is extremely rapid; hence, potential heat sinks such as large blood vessels have less of an impact compared to slower ablative techniques.

The oncological efficacy of HIFU is not fully determined. In the first phase 2 study of 18 tumors treated with HIFU and evaluated by subsequent nephrectomy, areas of coagulative necrosis comprised only 15% to 35% of the targeted tumor, indicating incomplete ablation (3). Illing et al treated eight renal tumors with another HIFU device (HAIFU). Four of six kidneys had radiographic evidence of successful ablation 12 days after the procedure, but histologic examination of four kidneys showed clear thermal damage in only one of the six kidneys (4).

The largest long-term study of HIFU involved a 3-year follow up of 17 patients treated with HIFU for renal masses with a mean size of 2.5 cm. There were no major complications related to HIFU and stable lesions were achieved in two-thirds of the patients (5). The difficulty in administering HIFU remains in energy attenuation by intervening tissue. While a laparoscopic approach is feasible, it detracts from the non-invasive advantage intrinsic to the extracorporeal approach. While limited data suggests HIFU to be inferior to existing ablative techniques, further studies are needed to determine patients that may benefit from this technology. Other minimally invasive technologies such as microwave thermotherapy and laser interstitial thermal therapy exist, but further long-term studies are needed to ascertain their role in the treatment of localized RCC.

NEAR-INFRARED FLUORESCENCE IMAGING

Near-infrared fluorescence (NIRF) imaging using intraoperative administration of indocyanine green (ICG) is another technology with emerging applications in urologic surgery. Due to preferential transport of ICG into proximal renal tubule cells, NIRF using intravenously injected ICG displays differential fluorescence in normal renal parenchyma compared to tumors and cysts. Theoretically, this imaging adjunct may assist in nephron-sparing surgery (NSS) where the desire is to preserve healthy tissue. The angiographic properties of ICG may also aid in the identification of renal vasculature and facilitate selective arterial clamping (6).

The two largest studies investigating the use of NIRF to aid in tumor localization have yielded inconsistent results. Manny et al described the ICG fluorescence pattern in 100 robot-assisted partial nephrectomies at a single institution (7). Hypofluoresence had both a high sensitivity and positive predictive value in determining malignant versus benign lesions. The authors concluded that ICG fluorescence patterns are associated with some histologic findings but are unable to reliably predict benign versus malignant lesions.

A standardized ICG dosing regimen was developed by Angel et al and achieved differential fluorescence in 82% of 79 tumors. Overall, 65 of 79 tumors behaved appropriately for an 86% agreement between histology and infrared fluorescence behavior (8). The greatest utility of NIRF may be in its ability to facilitate selective arterial clamping and aid in rapid identification of local perfusion deficits. Several recent studies have shown the decrease in global ischemia with selective arterial clamping using NIRF to minimize resultant loss of renal function (9–11).

> **KEY POINTS**
>
> 1. HIFU is an emerging alternative to RFA and cryoablation. Benefits include its noninvasive nature and rapid heat generation.
> 2. The oncologic efficacy of HIFU compared to traditional ablative techniques is currently unknown.
> 3. Intraoperative fluorescence imaging uses ICG to differentiate between various kidney tissue types.
> 4. While studies thus far have shown intraoperative fluorescence to be associated with characteristic histologic tumor, it is unable to reliably predict benign versus malignant lesions.
> 5. Intraoperative fluorescence may also permit selective arterial clamping and preservation of perioperative renal function.

REFERENCES

1. Whitson JM, Harris CR, Meng MV. Population-based comparative effectiveness of nephron-sparing surgery vs ablation for small renal masses. *BJU Int.* 2012;110(10):1438-1443.
2. Köhrmann KU, Michel MS, Gaa J, et al. High intensity focused ultrasound as noninvasive therapy for multilocal renal cell carcinoma: case study and review of the literature. *J Urol.* 2002;167(6):2397-2403.
3. Marberger M, Schatzl G, Cranston D, et al. Extracorporeal ablation of renal tumours with high-intensity focused ultrasound. *BJU Int.* 2005;95(Suppl 2):52-55.

4. Illing RO, Kennedy JE, Wu F, et al. The safety and feasibility of extracorporeal high-intensity focused ultrasound (HIFU) for the treatment of liver and kidney tumours in a Western population. *Br J Cancer.* 2005;93(8):890-895.
5. Ritchie RW, Leslie T, Phillips R, et al. Extracorporeal high intensity focused ultrasound for renal tumours: a 3-year follow-up. *BJU Int.* 2010;106(7):1004-1009.
6. Bjurlin MA, Gan M, McClintock TR, et al. Near-infrared fluorescence imaging: emerging applications in robotic upper urinary tract surgery. *Eur Urol.* 2014;65(4):793-801.
7. Manny TB, Krane LS, Hemal AK. Indocyanine green cannot predict malignancy in partial nephrectomy: histopathologic correlation with fluorescence pattern in 100 patients. *J Endourol.* 2013;27(7):918-921.
8. Angel JE, Khemees TA, Abaza R. Optimization of near infrared fluorescence tumor localization during robotic partial nephrectomy. *J Urol.* 2013;190(5):1668-1673.
9. Bjurlin MA, McClintock TR, Stifelman MD. Near-infrared fluorescence imaging with intraoperative administration of indocyanine green for robotic partial nephrectomy. *Curr Urol Rep.* 2015;16(4):20.
10. Borofsky MS, Gill IS, Hemal AK, et al. Near-infrared fluorescence imaging to facilitate super-selective arterial clamping during zero-ischaemia robotic partial nephrectomy. *BJU Int.* 2013;111(4):604-610.
11. Harke N, Schoen G, Schiefelbein F, et al. Selective clamping under the usage of near-infrared fluorescence imaging with indocyanine green in robot-assisted partial nephrectomy: a single-surgeon matched-pair study. *World J Urol.* 2014;32(5):1259-1265.

Kidney Cancer Survivorship Challenges and Issues 18

Elaine Chang and Wesley A. Mayer

RENAL DYSFUNCTION FOLLOWING NEPHRECTOMY

Renal dysfunction following nephrectomy is a recognized occurrence in survivors of cancer localized to the kidney. Mild decrease in glomerular filtration rate (GFR) is more common following radical nephrectomy than partial nephrectomy (1,2). Although nephrectomy in healthy patients does not result in clinically significant chronic renal impairment based on studies from kidney transplant donors, nephrectomy in patients with renal tumors involves a higher level of risk. In a retrospective study of patients with two healthy kidneys and normal serum creatinine (<1.4 mg/dL) who had elective partial or radical nephrectomy for a tumor that was 4 cm or smaller, the probability of new chronic kidney disease (CKD) (defined as GFR <60) at 3 years after surgery was **20%** after partial nephrectomy and **65%** after radical nephrectomy (1). In a separate retrospective study with a longer follow-up period that excluded patients with baseline CKD (creatinine >1.5 mg/dL), 22% of patients in the radical nephrectomy group experienced new onset CKD at 10 years, compared to 12% of patients in the nephron-sparing (partial nephrectomy) surgery group (2). However, conflicting data from a European randomized controlled trial in a similar patient population suggests that while more patients who receive radical nephrectomy compared to partial nephrectomy will subsequently experience GFR <60, the difference in the rate of patients who develop GFR <30 is not statistically significant between the 2 groups (3). In addition to the loss of functional nephrons, worsening of overall renal function may be attributed to the increase in GFR of the remaining nephrons, leading to hyperfiltration, an increase in glomerular pressure, and acceleration of preexisting renal disease (4). The rate of decrease in postoperative GFR in patients whose preoperative GFR is greater than 60 is widely variable in the literature.

Long-term surveillance for renal dysfunction includes following estimated GFR, quantification of any proteinuria, and review of urinalyses (5). While the gold standard for measurement of the GFR utilizes an infusion of inulin, estimation of filtration by the modification of diet in renal disease (MDRD) and Cockcroft-Gault formulas are often used for practical purposes. Proteinuria can be a marker of hyperfiltration and is associated with faster progression of CKD (2,5). This can be an indication for initiation of an angiotensin-converting-enzyme inhibitor or angiotensin receptor blocker, both of which can have renal protective effects.

LONG-TERM EFFECTS OF TARGETED AGENTS

Data on targeted agents thus far suggests that long-term effects should not be a routine concern.

- **Sorafenib**

  Evaluation of safety in patients with metastatic disease who received sorafenib for greater than 1 year in the phase 3 TARGET trial demonstrated no new toxic effects. Adverse effects were primarily grade 1 or 2, although 34% were grade 3 or 4. Most adverse effects, of any grade, developed in the first cycle and decreased in frequency with each subsequent cycle (6).

- **Sunitinib**

  Similarly, data from the global expanded access program for more than 4,500 patients who were treated with sunitinib for a median of 7 months, with 12 months of posttreatment follow-up, demonstrated that the safety profile appeared unchanged with long-term follow-up. Treatment schedule was 4 weeks on with two weeks off therapy prior to initiation of the next cycle. The three most common reasons for discontinuing therapy were lack of efficacy (39%), death (21%), and adverse effects (16%) (7).

- **Pazopanib**

  Long-term effects of pazopanib at 800 mg daily were studied in the extension study of the phase 3 placebo-controlled clinical trial. Median duration of treatment was 9.7 months, and 43% of patients received treatment for more than a year. The most common reason for discontinuation of therapy was progression of disease. The safety profile appeared unchanged compared to the original study in which median duration of treatment was 7.4 months, with the most common side effects being hypertension, diarrhea, hair color changes, and anorexia (8).

- **Axitinib**

  Pooled retrospective data of clinical trials utilizing single-agent axitinib at 5 mg twice daily demonstrated declining or stable rates of most adverse effects in patients who were treated for more than 2 years compared to those treated for shorter time periods. The exceptions were increasing amylase, and myocardial infarction, which increased from 0 during the initial 6 months of treatment to 3% and 5%, respectively, at 2 years (9).

SURVEILLANCE FOR CANCER RECURRENCE

After surgical excision of stage II or III disease, 20% to 40% of patients will experience relapse, the majority in the lungs. The optimal approach to postoperative surveillance is controversial. The American Urological Association (AUA) and National Comprehensive Cancer Network (NCCN) guidelines are the most widely referenced practice guidelines and are quite similar (10,11). They are displayed in Figures 18.1 and 18.2.

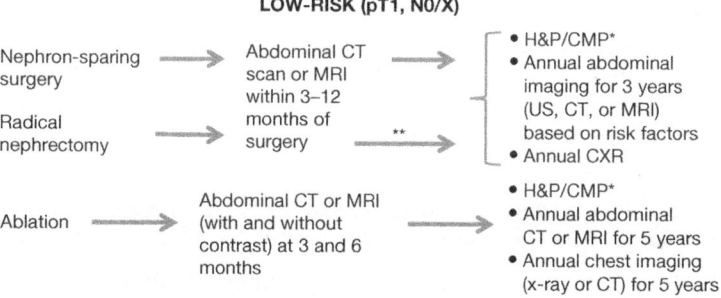

*NCCN recommends history & physical and CMP every 6 months for 2 years, and then annually for up to 5 years after nephrectomy (or diagnosis, in the case of ablation) (11).
**If the initial postoperative imaging after radical nephrectomy is negative, abdominal imaging beyond the first year may be performed at the clinician's discretion

Figure 18.1 AUA/NCCN guidelines for active surveillance after surgery in low-risk disease.

AUA, American Urological Association; CMP, comprehensive metabolic panel; CXR, chest x-ray; H&P, history and physical; NCCN, National Comprehensive Cancer Network; US, ultrasound.

120 KIDNEY CANCER

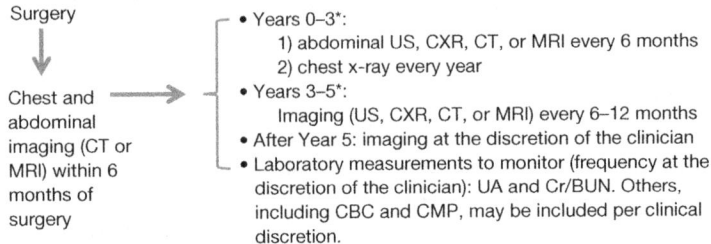

Figure 18.2 AUA/NCCN guidelines for active surveillance after surgery in moderate- to high-risk disease.

AUA, American Urological Association; BUN, blood urea nitrogen; CBC, complete blood count; CMP, comprehensive metabolic panel; Cr, creatinine; CXR, chest x-ray; NCCN, National Comprehensive Cancer Network; UA, urinalysis; US, ultrasound.

Some have suggested adjustments in screening depending on histologic subtype, based on observation of different recurrence patterns (12). The majority of clear cell tumors recur in the lungs, while the majority of papillary and chromophobe tumors recur within the abdomen. Additionally, the time to recurrence is significantly longer for chromophobe tumors (mean of 7 years, compared to a mean of 3.5–4 years in clear cell and papillary carcinomas). However, alternate screening algorithms have not yet been widely adopted.

KEY POINTS

- Patients are at risk for renal dysfunction following partial or radical nephrectomy.
- Targeted agents for metastatic disease are generally safe to use over the long term.
- Surveillance after curative intent surgery for kidney cancer should continue for up to five years.

REFERENCES

1. Huang WC, Levey AS, Serio AM, et al. Chronic kidney disease after nephrectomy in patients with renal cortical tumours: a retrospective cohort study. *Lancet Oncology.* 2006;7(9):735-740.
2. Lau WK, Blute ML, Weaver AL, et al. Matched comparison of radical nephrectomy vs nephron-sparing surgery in patients with unilateral renal cell carcinoma and a normal contralateral kidney. *Mayo Clin Proc.* 2000;75(12):1236-1242.
3. Scosyrev E, Messing EM, Sylvester R, et al. Renal function after nephron-sparing surgery versus radical nephrectomy: results from EORTC randomized trial 30904. *Eur Urol.* 2014;65(2):372-377.
4. Donckerwolcke RM, Coppes MJ. Adaptation of renal function after unilateral nephrectomy in children with renal tumours. *Pediatr Nephrol.* 2001;16:568-574.
5. Chapman D, Moore R, Klarenbach S, et al. Residual renal function after partial or radical nephrectomy for renal cell carcinoma. *Canadian Urol Assoc J.* 2010;4(5):337-343.
6. Hutson TE, Bellmunt J, Porta C, et al. Long-term safety of sorafenib in advanced renal cell carcinoma: follow-up of patients from phase III TARGET. *Eur J Cancer.* 2010;46(13):2432-2440.
7. Gore ME, Szczylik C, Porta C, et al. Final results from the large sunitinib global expanded-access trial in metastatic renal cell carcinoma. *Brit J Cancer.* 2015;113(1):12-19.
8. Sternberg CN, Davis ID, Deen KC, et al. An open-label extension study to evaluate safety and efficacy of pazopanib in patients with advanced renal cell carcinoma. *Oncol.* 2014;87(6):342-350.
9. Rini BI, Escudier B, Hariharan S, et al. Long-term safety with axitinib in previously treated patients with metastatic renal cell carcinoma. *Clin Genitourin Cancer.* 2015;13(6):540-547.
10. American Urological Association: Follow-up for clinically localized renal neoplasms: AUA guideline 2013. http://www.auanet.org/education/aua-guidelines.cfm
11. National Comprehensive Cancer Network. NCCN clinical practice guidelines in oncology: Kidney cancer 2.2016. http://www.nccn.org/professionals/ physician_gls/pdf/kidney.pdf
12. Siddiqui SA, Frank I, Cheville JC, et al. Postoperative surveillance for renal cell carcinoma: a multifactorial histological subtype specific protocol. *BJU Int.* 2009;104(6):778-785.

UPPER TRACT UROTHELIAL CANCER

Overview of Upper Tract Urothelial Cancers 19

Harish Madala, Carli Calderone, and Wesley A. Mayer

INTRODUCTION

Upper tract urothelial cancers (UTUC) include cancers arising from the urothelial lining anywhere between the renal calyces to the distal ureter. They are characterized by multifocality and share some similarities with urothelial carcinoma of the bladder. However, they tend to be much less common and pose a diagnostic challenge.

EPIDEMIOLOGY

UTUC involving the renal pelvis and ureter are relatively uncommon (5%–7% of all renal tumors). However, there is a higher incidence of UTUC in Balkan countries and Taiwan due to the specific risk factors (1,2).

The disease tends to be more common in White males, but disease-specific mortality rates are higher in African Americans and women (3). The mean age at diagnosis is 73, with peak incidence at 75 to 79 years. The incidence of renal pelvis tumors has been stable but the incidence of ureteral tumors has been steadily increasing, with a trend toward earlier stage at diagnosis. Multifocal involvement of the entire urinary tract is common, with 17% of patients having concurrent bladder tumors at presentation. The incidence of bilateral UTUC is 1.6%–6%.

ETIOLOGY

- Balkan nephropathy is a familial (but not hereditary) cause for multiple and bilateral UTUC cancers, which tend to be low grade. A possible association with dietary aristolochic acid consumption has been postulated. Surprisingly, bladder cancer incidence is unaffected (1).

- Smoking is the most important modifiable risk factor, with a 4- to 11-fold increased risk. The risk tends to be dose-related and declines after quitting, but never completely normalizes. Smokers are at increased risk for recurrence in the operative bed and have increased mortality (4).
- Phenacetin use with renal papillary necrosis has been associated with a 20-fold increased risk for UTUC together, but both are independent risk factors (5).
- There is increased incidence in Taiwan with artisan-well water use, which has high arsenic content. Arsenic-related UTUC is associated with increased mortality, but causality is yet to be identified (2).
- Hereditary UTUC has been noted to be associated with Lynch syndrome (6).
- The incidence of UTUC after prior bladder cancer is 2% to 4%. Factors that predict a higher risk for UTUC include grade, stage, TIS, multifocality, and tumors at the ureteral orifice. The incidence increases with bladder cancer follow-up duration. Patients with bladder carcinoma in situ (CIS) were noted to have more bilateral and lower ureteral involvement (7).

PRESENTATION

Signs and Symptoms

The most common presenting symptom of UTUC is hematuria, which is present at diagnosis in the majority of patients. This may be either grossly visible to the patient or microscopic on urinalysis (8). The patient may also complain of flank pain, although this is seen in less than half of cases. It is also possible for the patient to experience systemic "B" symptoms such as fever, night sweats, anorexia, weight loss, or fatigue. The presence of such symptoms should alert one to the increased possibility of metastatic disease (9).

Physical Examination, Laboratory Examination, and Imaging

On physical exam, an abdominal mass may be palpable in large tumors (8). In addition to microscopic hematuria, there may be decreased renal function in cases where the tumor is causing obstructive uropathy. While patients with normal contralateral renal function often compensate for obstruction, patients with the rare bilaterally obstructing tumors, solitary kidney, or chronic kidney disease will demonstrate a rise in creatinine. Imaging findings of hydronephrosis or a mass within the collecting system or the ureter could indicate UTUC. Although symptoms such as pain or presence of a mass are unrelated to prognosis, the presence of hydronephrosis is itself an independent indicator of more invasive disease (9,10).

DIAGNOSIS

Imaging

A CT urogram, which includes a delayed contrast phase in order to better visualize the collecting system, is the gold standard for assessing UTUC (11). It is between 67% and 100% sensitive and between 93% and 99% specific for detecting tumors in the collecting system and ureter (12). A reason for the high variability in sensitivity is due to decreased sensitivity in detecting CIS. This entity is flat and generally not visible on imaging, although urothelial thickening may be seen (13). CT is also used to assess for lymphadenopathy, which is highly predictive of metastatic disease in the context of UTUC (14). Hydronephrosis can also be assessed on CT urogram. Renal ultrasound can be used as a screening modality for obstruction (Figure 19.1a–c).

In cases where CT is contraindicated, MRI may be used; however the sensitivity of the exam decreases to 75% in tumors less than 2 cm (15). Additionally, one must use caution with gadolinium in patients with chronic kidney disease, as patients with a glomerular filtration rate (GFR) of less than 30 are at increased risk for nephrogenic systemic fibrosis.

126 UPPER TRACT UROTHELIAL CANCER

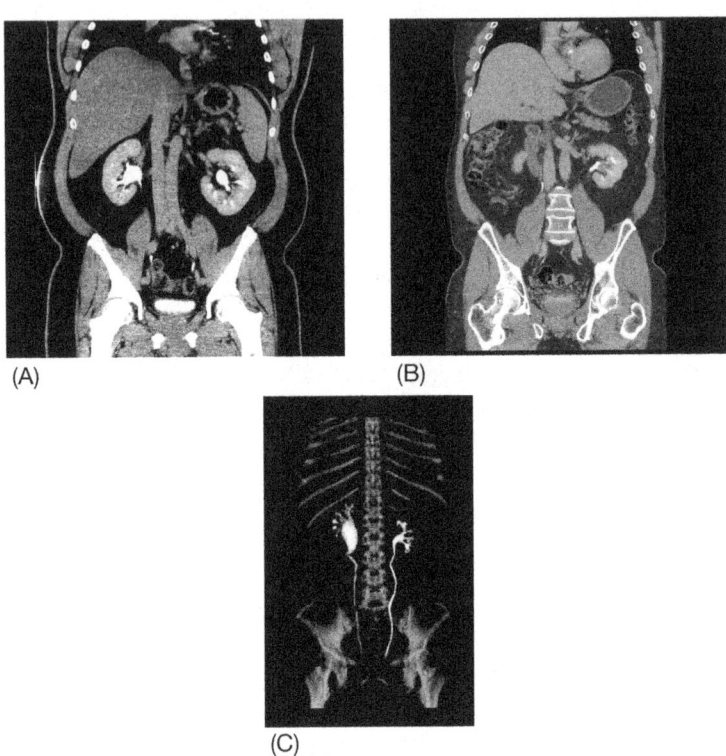

Figure 19.1 (A) Normal CT coronal urogram. (B) CT coronal showing a filling defect in the left collecting system corresponding to an upper tract high-grade urothelial carcinoma. (C) CT urogram reconstruction demonstrating a right UPJ obstruction from a kinking at the UPJ and a normal left collecting system and ureter.

UPJ, ureteropelvic junction.

Cytology and Tumor Markers

Cytology for UTUC is generally less sensitive than it is for bladder cancer. However, if UTUC is suspected, in situ washings of the collecting system should be performed in order to maximize diagnostic yield (16). The use of fluorescence in situ hybridization (FISH) seems to be more sensitive for UTUC than urine cytology (54% vs. 18% sensitive when bladder tumors were excluded) (17). However, it is still less sensitive than endoscopic evaluation and therefore has had little added value as a diagnostic tool.

Cystoscopy

Cystoscopy should always be performed in cases of UTUC to assess for concomitant bladder tumors (12). Positive urine cytology in the context of a negative cystoscopic exam might suggest UTUC, although CIS of the bladder is a possibility as well. Blue-light technology has increased our ability to detect flat lesions and might assist in detecting subtle bladder lesions, and will be discussed in more depth in Chapter 6A, Non Muscle Invasive Bladder Cancer.

In addition to direct visualization and biopsy of the bladder specimen, cystoscopy offers the opportunity to conduct retrograde pyelograms in order to further evaluate the upper tracts. Due to their high negative predictive value (92% vs. a 60% positive predictive value), they are particularly helpful in ruling out upper tract disease in cases where imaging is ambiguous (18). In the case of obstruction or poor visualization by this modality, percutaneous anterograde pyelograms may be considered. This method is preferred by some for larger tumors of the renal pelvis and proximal ureter (19).

Ureteroscopy

Ureteroscopy has demonstrated a higher sensitivity and specificity for the diagnosis of UTUC when compared with other methods, and is becoming the gold standard for diagnosis of UTUC (20). However, some clinicians may prefer to reserve ureteroscopy for times when management will be affected, such as when previous work-up is ambiguous or to avoid under-staging in the event that nephron-sparing management is being considered.

In addition to allowing for the direct visualization of upper tract lesions, ureteroscopy provides the opportunity for biopsy. Ureteroscopic biopsy is able to accurately determine tumor grade in greater than 90% of cases (20), although taken alone it is unreliable in the determination of tumor stage. Visualization is greatly aided by blue light technology, allowing for detection of flat lesions which would otherwise be missed (21,22). Ureteroscopy can also be used to collect in situ washings for cytology to increase yield in cases of CIS or otherwise difficult to visualize tumors (11).

Pathology

The majority (90%) of primary tumors arising in the renal pelvis and ureter are urothelial in origin. Squamous cell carcinoma makes up under 10% of these tumors, and less than 1% are adenocarcinoma (11). Small cell carcinoma has been described but is very rare.

Staging

Cancers of the upper tract urothelial area are staged using the tumor, node, metastasis (TNM) system (Table 19.1).

Table 19.1 Staging, American Joint Committee on Cancer, 8th Edition

	Primary tumor (T)
TX	Primary tumor cannot be assessed
T0	No evidence of primary tumor
Ta	Noninvasive papillary carcinoma
Tis	Carcinoma in situ
T1	Tumor invades subepithelial connective tissue
T2	Tumor invades muscularis
T3	Renal pelvis: tumor invades beyond muscularis into peripelvic fat or renal parenchyma; Ureter: tumor invades beyond muscularis into periureteric fat
T4	Tumor invades adjacent organs or through the kidney into perinephric fat
	Lymph nodes (N)
NX	Regional lymph nodes cannot be assessed
N0	No regional lymph node metastasis
N1	Metastasis in a single lymph node 2 cm or less in greatest dimension
N2	Metastasis in a single lymph node more than 2 cm; or multiple lymph nodes
	Distant metastasis (M)
M0	No distant metastasis
M1	Distant metastasis

Source: Adapted from Ref. (23). American Joint Committee on Cancer. Renal pelvis and ureter. In: Amin MB, Edge SB, Greene FL, et al., eds. *AJCC Cancer Staging Manual*. 8th ed. Chicago, IL: Springer; 2017:749-755.

Prognosis

Tumor stage is an important predictor of worse prognosis (Table 19.2).

Table 19.2 Survival Statistics	
Tumor stage	**5-year survival (%)**
pTa	64–100
pT1	75–92
pT2	72–83
pT3	41–62
pT4	0–41
Source: Adapted from Refs. (24–30).	

- **Stage:** Most important predictor of survival, with higher stage being indicative of a worse prognosis (31).
- **Grade:** Higher grade tumors are more likely to invade into the underlying structures and are associated with the presence of CIS (32).
- **Location:** Renal pelvis tumors generally have a better prognosis than ureteral cancers in terms of both recurrence-free and disease-specific survival in certain studies. Multifocality also predicts poor survival (33,34).
- **Lymphovascular invasion (LVI):** LVI has been shown to be an independent predictor of poor prognosis, with a higher risk for lymph node and distant metastases (35–37). It correlates well with the stage and grade of tumor. The 5-year survival rate for patients with LVI was 40% when compared to 80% in those without LVI (35).
- **Molecular markers:**
  a. *p53*: Overexpression of p53 has been associated with higher stage and worse prognosis, but it was not found to be an independent prognostic factor in multivariate analysis (25).
  b. *p27*: Decreased expression of p27 correlates with higher stage and lymph node metastases. However, it does not correlate with proliferation index or grade. It is associated with lower disease-free survival (DFS) but has no effect on overall survival (OS) (38).
  c. *Ki-67* index: It is associated with higher stage and grade UTUC as well as poor prognosis in terms of both DFS and OS (38).

d. Hypoxia inducible factor (HIF-1α): Higher levels are associated with higher T and N stage and is an independent predictor of decreased cancer-specific survival (39). Tumor necrosis also indicates worse prognosis (40).
- Miscellaneous: Preoperative CRP (40), low body mass index (34), and preoperative hydronephrosis (41) have also been associated with worse outcomes.

KEY POINTS

- While urothelial cancers involving the renal pelvis and ureter are relatively uncommon, they can be associated with bladder cancer in 17% of cases.
- Known risk factors include prior bladder cancer, Lynch syndrome, and exposure to aristolochic acid, tobacco, phenacetin, and arsenic.
- CT urogram is the gold standard for assessing upper tract urothelial carcinomas.
- Cystoscopy should always be performed in cases of UTUC to assess for concomitant bladder tumors.
- Ureteroscopy has high sensitivity and specificity for diagnosis and provides the opportunity to biopsy or obtain in situ washings.
- The most important predictor of outcome is higher stage, but other factors such as LVI, p53 overexpression, high Ki-67, high HIF-1α, and preoperative hydronephrosis may confer a worse prognosis.

REFERENCES

1. Grollman AP, Shibutani S, Moriya M, et al. Aristolochic acid and the etiology of endemic (Balkan) nephropathy. *Proc Nat Acad Sci.* 2007;104(29):12129-12134.
2. Tan LB, Chen KT, Guo-R. Clinical and epidemiological features of patients with genitourinary tract tumour in a blackfoot disease endemic area of Taiwan. *BJU Int.* 2008;102(1):48-54.
3. Munoz JJ, Ellison, LM. Upper tract urothelial neoplasms: incidence and survival during the last 2 decades. *J Urol.* 2000;164(5):1523-1525.

4. Van Osch SH, Jochems SH, van Schooten FJ, et al. Significant role for lifetime cigarette smoking in worsening bladder cancer and upper tract urothelial carcinoma prognosis: a meta-analysis. *J Urol.* 2016;195(4P1):872-879.
5. Ross RK, Paganini-Hill A, Landolph J, et al. Analgesics, cigarette smoking, and other risk factors for cancer of the renal pelvis and ureter. *Cancer Res.* 1989;49(4):1045-1048.
6. Rouprêt M, Yates DR, Comperat E, et al. Upper urinary tract urothelial cell carcinomas and other urological malignancies involved in the hereditary nonpolyposis colorectal cancer (lynch syndrome) tumor spectrum. *Eur Urol.* 2008;54(6):1226-1236.
7. Rabbani F, Perrotti M, Russo P, et al. Upper-tract tumors after an initial diagnosis of bladder cancer: Argument for long-term surveillance. *J Clin Oncol.* 2001;19(1):94-100.
8. Inman BA, Tran VT, Fradet Y, et al. Carcinoma of the upper urinary tract: predictors of survival and competing causes of mortality. *Cancer.* 2009;115(13):2853-2862.
9. Raman JD, Shariat SF, Karakiewicz PI, et al. Does preoperative symptom classification impact prognosis in patients with clinically localized upper-tract urothelial carcinoma managed by radical nephroureterectomy? *Urol Oncol.* 2011;29:716-723.
10. Messer JC, Terrell JD, Herman MP, et al. Multi-institutional validation of the ability of preoperative hydronephrosis to predict advanced pathologic tumor stage in upper-tract urothelial carcinoma. *Urol Oncol.* 2013;31(6):904-908.
11. Rouprêt M, Babjuk M, Böhle A, et al. Guidelines on urothelial carcinomas of the upper urinary tract. *Eur Assoc Urol.* 2015;68(5):1-21.
12. Cowan NC, Turney BW, Taylor NJ, et al. Multidetector computed tomography urography for diagnosing upper urinary tract urothelial tumour. *BJU Int.* 2007;99:1363-1370.
13. Xu AD, Ng CS, Kamat A, et al. Significance of upper urinary tract urothelial thickening and filling defect seen on MDCT urography in patients with a history of urothelial neoplasms. *AJR Am J Roentgenol.* 2010;195(4):959-965.
14. Millán-Rodríguez F, Palou J, de la Torre-Holguera P, et al. Conventional CT signs in staging transitional cell tumors of the upper urinary tract. *Eur Urol.* 1999;35(4):318-322.
15. Takahashi N, Glockner JF, Hartman RP, et al. Gadolinium enhanced magnetic resonance urography for upper urinary tract malignancy. *J Urol.* 2010;183(4):1330-1365.
16. Messer J, Shariat SF, Brien JC, et al. Urinary cytology has a poor performance for predicting invasive or high-grade upper-tract urothelial carcinoma. *BJU Int.* 2011;108(5):701-705.
17. Johannes JR, Nelson E, Bibbo M, et al. Voided urine fluorescence in situ hybridization testing for upper tract urothelial carcinoma surveillance. *J Urol.* 2010;184(3):879-882.

18. Lee KS, Zeikus E, DeWolf WC, et al. MR urography versus retrograde pyelography/ureteroscopy for the exclusion of upper urinary tract malignancy. *Clin Radiol.* 2010;65:185-192.
19. Raman JD, Scherr DS. Management of patients with upper urinary tract transitional cell carcinoma. *Nat Clin Pract Urol.* 2007;4:432-443.
20. Rojas CP, Castle SM, Llanos CA, et al. Low biopsy volume in ureteroscopy does not affect tumor biopsy grading in upper tract urothelial carcinoma. *Urol Oncol.* 2013;31(8):1696-1700.
21. Stenzl A, Burger M, Fradet Y, et al. Hexaminolevulinate guided fluorescence cystoscopy reduces recurrence in patients with non-muscle invasive bladder cancer. *J Urol.* 2010;184(5):1907-1913.
22. Ray ER, Chatterton K, Khan MS, et al. Hexylaminolaevulinate 'blue light' fluorescence cystoscopy in the investigation of clinically unconfirmed positive urine cytology. *BJU Int.* 2009;103:1363-1367.
23. American Joint Committee on Cancer. Renal pelvis and ureter. In: Amin MB, Edge SB, Greene FL, et al., eds. *AJCC Cancer Staging Manual.* 8th ed. Chicago, IL: Springer; 2017:749-755.
24. Corrado F, Ferri C, Mannini D, et al. Transitional cell carcinoma of the upper urinary tract: evaluation of prognostic factors by histopathology and flow cytometric analysis. *J Urol.* 1991;145:1159-1163.
25. Rey A, Lara PC, Redondo E, et al. Overexpression of p53 in transitional cell carcinoma of the renal pelvis and ureter. *Cancer.* 1997;79:2178-2185.
26. Masuda M, Iki M, Takano Y, et al. Prognostic significance of Ki-67 labeling index in urothelial tumors of the renal pelvis and ureter. *J Urol.* 1996;155:1877-1881.
27. Hall MC, Womack S, Sagalowsky AI, et al. Prognostic factors, recurrence, and survival in transitional cell carcinoma of the upper urinary tract: a 30-year experience in 252 patients. *Urol.* 1998;52:594-601.
28. Morioka M, Jo Y, Furukawa Y, et al. Prognostic factors for survival and bladder recurrence in transitional cell carcinoma of the upper urinary tract. *Int J Urol.* 2001;8:30-37.
29. Kirkali Z, Moffat LEF, Deane RF, et al. Urothelial tumours of the upper urinary tract. *Br J Urol.* 1989;64:18-24.
30. Mufti GR, Gove JRW, Badenoch DF, et al. Transitional cell carcinoma of the renal pelvis and ureter. *Br J Urol.* 1989;63:135-140.
31. Png KS, Lim EK., Chong, KT, et al. Prognostic factors for upper tract transitional cell carcinoma: a retrospective review of 66 patients. *Asian J Surg.* 2008;31(1):20-24.
32. Epstein JI, Amin MB, Reuter VR, et al. The World Health Organization/International Society of Urological Pathology consensus classification of urothelial (transitional cell) neoplasms of the urinary bladder. *Am J Surg Pathol.* 1998;22(12):1435-1448.

33. Park S, Hong B, Kim C, et al. The impact of tumor location on prognosis of transitional cell carcinoma of the upper urinary tract. *J Urol*. 2004;171(2):621-625.
34. Kang HW, Jung HD, Ha YS, et al. Preoperative underweight patients with upper tract urothelial carcinoma survive less after radical nephroureterectomy. *J Korean Med Sci*. 2015;30(10):1483-1489.
35. Kikuchi E, Horiguchi Y, Nakashima J, et al. Lymphovascular invasion independently predicts increased disease specific survival in patients with transitional cell carcinoma of the upper urinary tract. *J Urol*. 2005;174(6):2120-2124.
36. Lin WC, Hu FC, Chung SD, et al. The role of lymphovascular invasion in predicting the prognosis of clinically localized upper tract urothelial carcinoma (pT1-3cN0M0). *J Urol*. 2008;180(3):879-885.
37. Saito K, Kawakami S, Fujii Y, et al. Lymphovascular invasion is independently associated with poor prognosis in patients with localized upper urinary tract urothelial carcinoma treated surgically. *J Urol*. 2007;178(6):2291-2296.
38. Kamai T, Takagi K, Asami H, et al. Prognostic significance of p27Kip1 and Ki-67 expression in carcinoma of the renal pelvis and ureter. *BJU Int*. 2000;86(1):14-19.
39. Ke HL, Wei YC, Yang SF, et al. Overexpression of hypoxia-inducible factor-1α predicts an unfavorable outcome in urothelial carcinoma of the upper urinary tract. *Int J Urol*. 2008;15(3):200-205.
40. Luo Y, Fu SJ, She DL, et al. Preoperative C-reactive protein as a prognostic predictor for upper tract urothelial carcinoma: a systematic review and meta-analysis. *Mol Clin Oncol*. 2015;3(4):924-928.
41. Yeh HC, Jan HC, Wu WJ, et al. Concurrent preoperative presence of hydronephrosis and flank pain independently predicts worse outcome of upper tract urothelial carcinoma. *PLoS One*. 2015;10(10):e0139624.

Management of Early Stage Upper Tract Urothelial Cancers 20

Harish Madala, Carli Calderone, and Wesley A. Mayer

INTRODUCTION

Surgical management of upper urothelial tract cancers (UTUC) includes both nephron-sparing approaches and radical nephroureterectomy (RNU) with lymph node dissection (LND). Patients with UTUC must first be stratified into low risk and high risk in order to determine the appropriate therapy.

In order to be considered low risk, a tumor must comply with *all* of the following criteria: unifocal, small (<1 cm), low grade on both cytology and ureteroscopic biopsy, and have no evidence of infiltrative disease on CT urogram. In contrast, any one of the following features of a tumor constitutes high risk: the presence of hydronephrosis, large (>1 cm), high grade by either cytology or ureteroscopic biopsy, multifocal tumors, or UTUC occurring after radical cystectomy for bladder cancer (Table 20.1).

Table 20.1 Risk Stratification

Low risk	High risk*
Unifocal	Multifocal
Size: <1 cm	Size: >1 cm
Low-grade histology on cytology or biopsy	High-grade histology on cytology or biopsy
No evidence of infiltrative disease on CTU	Presence of hydronephrosis
	UTUC occurring after radical cystectomy for bladder cancer
CTU, CT urogram; UTUC, upper tract urothelial cancer.	
*Note: If any single high-risk feature is present, tumor is considered to be high risk.	

NEPHRON-SPARING SURGICAL APPROACHES

There are two populations of patients for which nephron-sparing management may be appropriate. Nephron-sparing approaches should be considered in all cases of low-risk disease (1). Candidates must be counseled extensively on the need for stringent follow-up after surgery and be willing and able to comply. Otherwise, more aggressive therapy should be considered.

Nephron-sparing procedures may also be necessary in the case of high-risk disease where the contralateral kidney is compromised, as is the case with chronic kidney disease, or in patients with solitary kidneys. Cases must be evaluated on an individual basis according to the patient's comorbidities, life expectancy, compliance, and preferences.

Endoscopic laser ablation is appropriate for low-risk tumors (1). This is generally accomplished ureteroscopically; however, percutaneous access may be necessary if tumor is inaccessible from a retrograde approach or due to tumor size. Although the percutaneous approach is being utilized less as ureteroscopic techniques and instrumentation advance, it is still a very important approach for some patients (2).

Segmental ureteral resection is indicated in the case of endoscopic failure to remove low-risk tumors, or for all high-risk tumors of the distal ureter when nephron-sparing management is chosen. When high-risk tumors meet certain criteria, the cancer control and survival has been found to be similar between segmental resection and RNU; these characteristics include unifocal tumors of the distal ureter less than 2 cm and ≤ stage T2 (3). Previous research has found that iliac or lumbar ureteral resection may have a higher failure rate than distal ureteral resection (1). Thus, tumor location may play a key role in determining candidacy for nephron-sparing management of high-risk tumors. Lymphadenectomy can also be performed as a part of segmental ureteral resection, and is indicated on a case-by-case basis in instances of high-grade tumor (3).

Radical Nephroureterectomy

In patients with high-risk disease, or in patients who are not able to meet the surveillance requirements of conservative management, a RNU with excision of the bladder cuff is the gold standard of treatment. When comparing laparoscopic versus open techniques for RNU, multiple retrospective studies have generally found them to have comparable oncologic outcomes (4–7). Because open RNU is generally offered to patients who are at the highest risk, a question of selection bias has arisen. Regardless, laparoscopic approaches are being increasingly utilized and are generally accepted to provide adequate cancer control.

Robotic approaches have been introduced over the last decade. Sufficient long-term data are still lacking; however, early and intermediate cancer control has been shown to be on par with that of open and laparoscopic approaches (6). A single randomized controlled trial (RCT) demonstrated similar oncologic outcomes between the two approaches in patients with organ-confined disease, with the robotic group experiencing less blood loss and a shorter length of stay (7).

Lymph Node Dissections

There is an insufficient amount of data about the oncologic implications of performing LNDs in patients with UTUC, and thus the topic remains highly debated. However, it is generally thought to be unnecessary to perform an LND on Ta and T1 disease, as the yield of positive nodes is low. Positive lymph nodes are found in 2.2% of patients with Ta or T1 disease compared to 16% in disease staged T2 or greater (8). For T2 disease and above, surgeons generally follow an LND template rather than strive to obtain a specific number of nodes, which does correlate to improved survival (9).

Adjuvant Therapy

Bacillus Calmette-Guérin (BCG) instillation for early/limited stage UTUC has historically not shown any survival benefit (10). However, it may have some role in renal preservation and improving quality of life, especially in patients with carcinoma *in situ* (11). There is a risk for sepsis if instilled at high pressures or in a patient with an active urinary tract infection.

High-risk patients may benefit from postoperative intravesical chemotherapy to reduce bladder recurrence (12–15).

Systemic chemotherapy has not shown benefit in early stage UTUC (16).

Surveillance

Recurrence can be local or distant. Any recurrence in the upper tract or bladder itself is considered local (17). Local recurrence is seen most commonly after nephron-sparing management, and is less common after RNU, where most recurrences are in the form of metastases. As such, follow-up schedules and modalities vary by treatment approach and are discussed as follows.

Post-RNU

Local recurrence is very rare after RNU; however, it is recommended to perform cystoscopy and urine cytology at 3 months after surgery and annually after that for at least 5 years. The risk of distant metastases is related to the features of the tumor. For noninvasive tumors, a CT urogram should be obtained annually for at least 5 years. For invasive tumors, a CT urogram should be obtained every 6 months for the first 2 years, and then annually for a total of at least 5 years.

After Nephron-Sparing Treatment

As previously mentioned, nephron-sparing approaches require much more rigorous follow-up; therefore, patient selection is of utmost importance. CT urogram and urine cytology should be performed at 3 months, 6 months, and then annually for at least 5 years. Special consideration may be given to patients with chronic kidney disease (CKD), who cannot receive contrast needed for a CT urogram. Additionally for high-risk patients, cystoscopy, ureteroscopy, and cytology in situ should be performed at 3 months, 6 months, then every 6 months for 2 years, and then annually for a total of at least 5 years. Recurrence rates decrease over time, so early follow-up is essential in detecting tumors, especially those that may have been understaged (18).

KEY POINTS

- Nephron-sparing surgery should be considered in all cases of low-risk disease.
- Segmental ureteral resection is an option in the case of endoscopic failure to remove low-risk tumors.
- In high-risk disease, RNU with excision of the bladder cuff is the gold standard. Nephron-sparing surgery may be necessary when the contralateral kidney is compromised.
- Oncologic outcomes may be equivalent with open surgery, laparoscopic approaches, and robotic approaches, but sufficient long-term data are not yet available.
- Long-term follow up is essential after surgical management.

REFERENCES

1. Rouprêt M, Babjuk M, Böhle A, et al. Guidelines on urothelial carcinomas of the upper urinary tract. *Eur Assoc Urol.* 2015; 68(5):1-21.
2. Rouprêt M, Traxer O, Tligui M, et al. Upper urinary tract transitional cell carcinoma: recurrence rate after percutaneous endoscopic resection. *Eur Urol.* 2007;51:709-714.
3. Colin P, Ouzzane A, Pignot G, et al. Comparison of oncological outcomes after segmental ureterectomy or radical nephroureterectomy in urothelial carcinomas of the upper urinary tract: results from a large French multicentre study. *BJU Int.* 2012;110:1134-1141.
4. Ni S, Tao W, Chen Q, et al. Laparoscopic versus open nephroureterectomy for the treatment of upper urinary tract urothelial carcinoma: a systematic review and cumulative analysis of comparative studies. *Eur Urol.* 2012;61:1142-1153.
5. Capitanio U, Shariat SF, Isbarn H, et al. Comparison of oncologic outcomes for open and laparoscopic nephroureterectomy: a multi-institutional analysis of 1249 cases. *Eur Urol.* 2009;56:1-9.
6. Aboumohamed AA, Krane LS, Hemal AK. Oncologic outcomes following robot-assisted laparoscopic nephroureterectomy with bladder cuff excision for upper tract urothelial carcinoma. *J Urol.* 2015;194:1561-1566.
7. Simone G, Papalia R, Guaglianone S, et al. Laparoscopic versus open nephroureterectomy: perioperative and oncologic outcomes from a randomised prospective study. *Eur Urol.* 2009;56:520-526.

8. Fajkovic H, Cha EK, Jeldres C, et al. Prognostic value of extranodal extension and other lymph node parameters in patients with upper tract urothelial carcinoma. *J Urol.* 2012;187:845-851.
9. Kondo T, Hashimoto Y, Kobayashi H, et al. Template-based lymphadenectomy in urothelial carcinoma of the upper urinary tract: Impact on patient survival. *Int J Urol.* 2012;17:848-854.
10. Rastinehad AR, Ost MC, Vanderbrink BA, et al. A 20-year experience with percutaneous resection of upper tract transitional carcinoma: is there an oncologic benefit with adjuvant bacillus Calmette Guérin therapy? *Urol.* 2009;73(1):27-31.
11. Giannarini G, Kessler TM, Birkhäuser FD, et al. Antegrade perfusion with bacillus Calmette-Guérin in patients with non–muscle-invasive urothelial carcinoma of the upper urinary tract: who may benefit? *Eur Urol.* 2011;60(5):955-960.
12. Rouprêt M, Babjuk M, Böhle A, et al. European Association of Urology guidelines on upper urinary tract urothelial cell carcinoma: 2015 update. *Eur Urol.* 2015;68(5):868-879.
13. O'Brien T, Ray E, Singh R, et al. Prevention of bladder tumours after nephroureterectomy for primary upper urinary tract urothelial carcinoma: a prospective, multicentre, randomised clinical trial of a single postoperative intravesical dose of Mitomycin C (the ODMIT-C Trial). *Eur Urol.* 2011;60(4):703-710.
14. Fang D, Li XS, Xiong GY, et al. Prophylactic intravesical chemotherapy to prevent bladder tumors after nephroureterectomy for primary upper urinary tract urothelial carcinomas: a systematic review and meta-analysis. *Urol Int.* 2013;91(3):291-296.
15. Ito A, Shintaku I, Satoh M, et al. Prospective randomized phase II trial of a single early intravesical instillation of pirarubicin (THP) in the prevention of bladder recurrence after nephroureterectomy for upper urinary tract urothelial carcinoma: the THP Monotherapy Study Group Trial. *J Clin Oncol.* 2013;31(11):1422-1427.
16. Hellenthal NJ, Shariat SF, Margulis V, et al. Adjuvant chemotherapy for high risk upper tract urothelial carcinoma: results from the Upper Tract Urothelial Carcinoma Collaboration. *J Urol.* 2009;182(3):900-906.
17. Seisen T, Granger B, Colin P, et al. A systematic review and meta-analysis of clinicopathologic factors linked to intravesical recurrence after radical nephroureterectomy to treat upper tract urothelial carcinoma. *Eur Urol.* 2015;67:1122-1133.
18. Colin P, Ghoneim TP, Nison L, et al. Risk stratification of metastatic recurrence in invasive upper urinary tract carcinoma after radical nephroureterectomy without lymphadenectomy. *World J Urol.* 2013;32:507-512.

Treatment of Metastatic Upper Tract Urothelial Cancers 21

Jose Pacheco, Saleha Sajid, and Teresa Gray Hayes

FIRST-LINE CHEMOTHERAPY OPTIONS

Urothelial carcinoma (UC) of the upper tract is a rare, aggressive urologic cancer with a tendency to metastasize early. Level 1 evidence from a prospective randomized controlled trial (RCT) is not available given its rarity, and treatment strategies are adapted from metastatic UC of the bladder (Chapter 26). The two first-line chemotherapy options in patients with good organ function and performance status (Eastern Cooperative Oncology Groups Performance Status 0 to 1) are gemcitabine plus cisplatin (GC) and dose-dense methotrexate + vinblastine + adriamycin + cisplatin (ddMVAC) (Table 21.1). However, a direct comparison between GC and ddMVAC has not been done in a randomized trial. The phase 3 multicenter RCT that suggested similar survival and a more tolerable side effect profile for GC (significantly less grade 3/4 neutropenia, neutropenic fever, neutropenic sepsis, mucositis, and alopecia) was comparing it to standard MVAC (sMVAC) (1). The reasons why ddMVAC is preferred in clinical practice over sMVAC are 3-fold based on the results of an RCT in metastatic UC of the bladder:

i. ddMVAC demonstrated an improved overall response rate (ORR) compared to sMVAC (64% vs. 50%) and improved progression free survival (PFS) (9.5 months vs. 8.1 months)
ii. While there was no significant difference in median overall survival (OS), the 5-year OS was significantly better for ddMVAC at 21.8% versus 13.5% with sMVAC
iii. ddMVAC was better tolerated than sMVAC with less grade 3 to 4 leukopenia, neutropenic fever, and mucositis (2)

Table 21.1 First-Line Regimens for Advanced Urothelial Carcinoma		
Cisplatin eligible	**Cisplatin ineligible**[a,b]	**If Her2 positive**
a. ddMVAC b. GC	a. Carboplatin-based regimens b. Taxol-based regimens c. Single agent chemotherapy regimens d. Clinical trial e. Can consider atezolizumab, nivolumab, or another immune checkpoint inhibitor*	a. Can consider clinical trials of Her2 targeting agent alone or in combination with chemotherapy
ddMVAC, dose-dense methotrexate + vinblastine + adriamycin + cisplatin; GC, gemcitabine + cisplatin. [a]Ineligibility criteria for cisplatin include: creatinine clearance less than 60 mL/min by the Cockcroft Gault formula, ECOG PS $\geq$ 2, grade $\geq$ 2 hearing loss, and grade $\geq$ 2 peripheral neuropathy. [b]For select patients with creatinine clearance between 45 and 59 mL/min by the Cockcroft Gault formula, one can consider split dose cisplatin-based regimens. *Immune checkpoint inhibitors have not been approved at the time of this publication for first-line therapy in cisplatin ineligible patients with metastatic urothelial cancer. However, several of them are undergoing Federal Drug Administration review for this indication and are likely to be approved soon.		

It is unclear if efficacy can be preserved in metastatic UC when carboplatin is substituted for cisplatin. Such a substitution is not currently recommended if a patient can tolerate cisplatin (3).

FIRST-LINE CHEMOTHERAPY OPTIONS IN HER2-POSITIVE CANCER

Her2 is overexpressed 3+ by immunohistochemistry or $\geq$ 2.2 by fluorescence in situ hybridization in some cases of UC. Estimates of overexpression in urothelial tumors range from 5% to 81%, with the majority of tested primaries being of bladder origin and average overexpression being about 16% when taking into account most published studies. A randomized phase 2 study suggested possible benefit when trastuzumab was combined with GC in UC overexpressing Her2; however, further randomized trials comparing combination chemotherapy including trastuzumab to the current standards of care (GC or ddMVAC) must be conducted before trastuzumab gains an established role in the upfront setting for Her2-overexpressing metastatic UC (4). Other Her2-targeted agents have shown efficacy in select patient populations; however, the data are still premature.

The use of trastuzumab or other targeted agents that inhibit Her2 are not currently part of the National Comprehensive Cancer Network (NCCN) Clinical Practice Guidelines in Oncology (NCCN Guidelines®) (5).

FIRST-LINE CHEMOTHERAPY OPTIONS WITH CREATININE CLEARANCE LESS THAN 60 ML/MIN

One option would be to split the dose of cisplatin, giving half the dose on day 1 and the other half on day 2 of each cycle. This is generally only done when the creatinine clearance (CrCl) is between 45 and 60 mL/min (6). Administering split-dose cisplatin as part of GC is a common clinical practice; however, it is not part of the NCCN Guidelines in the metastatic setting due to limited data. In such patients, the NCCN recommends as category 2B options carboplatin- or taxol-based combinations or single-agent chemotherapy. Additionally, one can consider clinical trials (Table 21.1) (5). However, one must be aware that combination regimens have poor efficacy when both the CrCl is less than 60 mL/min and the Eastern Cooperative Oncology Group Performance Status is ≥ 2.

Published results of cohort 1 of the IMvigor210 study suggest that atezolizumab may be efficacious in patients who are not eligible for first-line platinum-based therapy. With 17.2 months median follow-up, patients treated with atezolizumab had a median OS of 15.9 months, which was better than historical controls, who had a median OS of 9 to 10 months (7). These encouraging results must be replicated in a phase 3 RCT before atezolizumab becomes part of routine care in this setting. However, it may become a future standard in patients ineligible for first-line cisplatin-based combination chemotherapy (Table 21.1).

GC PLUS BEVACIZUMAB IN METASTATIC UROTHELIAL CANCER

The use of GC plus bevacizumab has been evaluated in a phase 2 clinical trial exploring a first-line regimen for metastatic UC. In this study, the ORR was 72%, median PFS was 8.2 months, and median OS was 19.1 months. Significant grade 3 to 4 toxicities included neutropenia (35%) and thromboembolism (21%). The primary endpoint of a 50% improvement in PFS compared to historical controls (7.5 months) was not met (8). Larger scale, randomized clinical trials need to be conducted to reproduce these results before this regimen is widely implemented.

Due to similar recommendations for metastatic UC of the bladder, regimens in the second-line setting and beyond will be discussed Chapter 26.

KEY POINTS

- First-line regimens with category 1 recommendations for metastatic UC are GC and ddMVAC.
- There is a lack of data to support substituting carboplatin for cisplatin in patients who are eligible for cisplatin-based therapy.
- In patients with CrCl less than 60 mL/min, one may consider combination chemotherapy with split-dose cisplatin, carboplatin- or taxol-based combinations, or single-agent regimens.

REFERENCES

1. von der Maase H, Hansen SW, Roberts JT, et al. Gemcitabine and cisplatin versus methotrexate, vinblastine, doxorubicin, and cisplatin in advanced or metastatic bladder cancer: results of a large, randomized, multinational, multicenter, phase III study. *J Clin Oncol.* 2000;18(17):3068-3077.
2. Sternberg CN, de Mulder PH, Schornagel JH, et al. Seven year update of an EORTC phase III trial of high-dose intensity M-VAC chemotherapy and G-CSF versus classic M-VAC in advanced urothelial tract tumors. *Eur J Cancer.* 2006;41(1):50-54.

3. Garcia JA, Dreicer R. Systemic chemotherapy for advanced bladder cancer: update and controversies. *J Clin Oncol.* 2006;24(35):5545-5551.
4. Oudard S, Culine S, Vano Y, et al. Multicentre randomized phase 2 trial of gemcitabine + platinum, with or without trastuzumab, in advanced or metastatic urothelial carcinoma overexpressing Her2. *Eur J Cancer.* 2015;51(1):45-54.
5. Bladder Cancer Guidelines Version 2.2017. Referenced with permission from the NCCN Clinical Practice Guidelines in Oncology (NCCN Guidelines®) for Bladder Cancer V.2.2017. © National Comprehensive Cancer Network, Inc. 2017. All rights reserved. Accessed [March 22, 2017]. To view the most recent and complete version of the guideline, go online to NCCN.org. NATIONAL COMPREHENSIVE CANCER NETWORK®, NCCN®, NCCN GUIDELINES®, and all other NCCN Content are trademarks owned by the National Comprehensive Cancer Network, Inc.
6. Galsky MD, Hahn NM, Rosenberg J, et al. Treatment of patients with metastatic urothelial cancer "unfit" for cisplatin-based chemotherapy. *J Clin Oncol.* 2011;29(17):2432-2438.
7. Balar AV, Galsky MD, Rosenberg JE, et al. Atezolizumab as first-line treatment in cisplatin-ineligible patients with locally advanced and metastatic urothelial carcinoma: a single-arm, multi-centre, phase 2 trial. *Lancet.* 2017;389(10064):67-76.
8. Hahn NM, Stadler WM, Zon RT, et al. Phase II trial of cisplatin, gemcitabine, and bevacizumab as first-line therapy for metastatic urothelial carcinoma: Hoosier Oncology Group GU-04-75. *J Clin Oncol.* 2011;29(12):1525-1530.

Controversies in the Management of Upper Tract Urothelial Cancer 22

Jose Pacheco and Jennifer Marie Taylor

Case 1: A 53-year-old male presented with a right renal mass that was 21.2 cm in maximal diameter, with ipsilateral hydronephrosis, a 1 cm hepatic lesion, and bilateral sub-centimeter pulmonary nodules. He had a ureteroscopic biopsy that showed papillary urothelial carcinoma.

Question 1: Is surgery an option for this patient?
For metastatic renal cell carcinoma (RCC), cytoreductive nephrectomy has been shown to have a survival benefit. Since some upper tract urothelial cancers (UTUC) have a similar location and pattern of spread as RCC, one could hypothesize that some patients with these tumors may also benefit from cytoreductive surgery.

Unfortunately, there are no randomized trials examining cytoreductive surgery and/or metastatectomy in UTUC. However, there are retrospective studies evaluating the benefit of surgery in metastatic urothelial cancer, in which UTUC cases comprise 20% to 56% in the cohorts (1–4). In these retrospective studies there is suggestion that some patients may benefit from surgery (Table 22.1).

With lack of randomized controlled trials or robust retrospective data, the question of surgery in metastatic UTUC is controversial. However, the question may arise in select cases, especially those who have no comorbidities and a limited metastatic burden. Some experts advocate chemotherapy followed by surgical intervention only if clinical downstaging is seen radiographically. Retrospective data do seem to suggest some benefit to metastatectomy in cases with limited metastasis, but the benefit of cytoreductive surgery without metastatectomy is not known. Intervention in this setting must be in carefully selected patients who understand the limited known benefit.

Table 22.1 Retrospective Studies of Metastatectomy in Metastatic Urothelial Cancer

Study	Patients (n)	Upper urothelial tract tumors (n)	Resected sites	Median time to recurrence (months)	PFS	OS	Type of surgery	Systemic treatment
Abe et al. (1)	42	18	19%—Regional lymph nodes 29%—Distant lymph nodes 2.4%—Bone 40%—Visceral 12%—Local recurrence	N/A	N/A	5-y OS—31%	Metastatectomy	81% NA chemotherapy 17% A chemotherapy
Bekku et al. (2)	27	15	17%—Lung 83%—Retroperitoneal lymph nodes	N/A	12 patients with PR and surgery—3-y PFS 40% 15 patients with PR and no surgery—3-y PFS 0%	3-y OS in those with PR and surgery—72% 3-y OS in those with PR and no surgery—12%	Metastatectomy	100% NA chemotherapy

(continued)

Table 22.1 Retrospective Studies of Metastatectomy in Metastatic Urothelial Cancer (continued)

Study	Patients (n)	Upper urothelial tract tumors (n)	Resected sites	Median time to recurrence (months)	PFS	OS	Type of surgery	Systemic treatment
Lehman et al. (3)	44	9	56.8%—Retroperitoneal lymph nodes 11.3%—Distant lymph nodes 4.5%—Bone 9.2%—Visceral	N/A	5 y—24%	5 y—28%	Metastatectomy	50% NA chemotherapy 43% A chemotherapy
Siefker-Radtke et al. (4)	31	7	87%—Visceral (77% lung) 13%—Distant lymph nodes	7	N/A	5-y OS 33%	Metastatectomy	71% NA chemotherapy 29% A chemotherapy

A, adjuvant; N/A, not available; NA, neoadjuvant; OS, overall survival; PFS, progression free survival; PR, partial response.

Source: Adapted from Refs. (1, 2, 3, 4)

Case 2: A 53-year old underwent a radical nephroureterectomy and lymph node dissection (LND) for a urothelial carcinoma of the renal pelvis. He completed 4 cycles of adjuvant Gemcitabine + Cisplatin. One year later he was noted to have a 2 cm left lower lobe lung nodule. Biopsy of this lesion was consistent with urothelial cell carcinoma. On CT imaging of the chest/abdomen/pelvis there were no other sites of disease.

Question 2: Should this patient undergo resection of the lung nodule?

Metastatectomy appears to have some survival benefit in limited retrospective studies, some of which were discussed earlier in this section. Those most likely to benefit from such an approach are those with small volume metastasis (e.g., isolated visceral metastasis or nodal metastasis) and in the context of chemotherapy (5). However, this is a controversial issue that will require further analysis as there are inherent biases in retrospective studies, including small case numbers and lack of generalizability. Metastatectomy may be considered in select cases, but it should not be widely adapted in the community without further data, preferably via randomized or multicenter prospective studies. Randomized studies remain quite hard to accrue in a disease as rare as UTUC, but multicenter cooperative group efforts can potentially provide future answers to questions like this.

Question 3: Should this patient undergo neoadjuvant therapy before resection of the lung metastasis or adjuvant therapy afterwards?

Some experts have argued that neoadjuvant chemotherapy should be given prior to metastatectomy. The rationale behind this approach is that it allows the treating physicians to see who will and will not respond to chemotherapy. Those who respond are the ones who obtain the benefit from metastatectomy in the published retrospective trials (5).

Case 3: A 63-year-old male patient undergoes imaging and endoscopic diagnosis to confirm a high-grade 4 cm renal pelvis tumor. Depth of invasion is difficult to determine due to bulk of tumor in the renal pelvis. Staging imaging shows no evidence of lymphatic or distant metastasis, and his estimated glomerular filtration rate (eGFR) is greater than 60.

Question 4: What is the preferred sequence of definitive treatment?

Although no level 1 evidence provides the answer to this question, the current recommendation, being tested in prospective studies, is for the patient to receive neoadjuvant cisplatin-based chemotherapy followed by radical nephroureterectomy with regional LND. Limited retrospective data support this approach (6). The most important reasons for this are the known rates of clinical understaging of upper tract primary lesions and the expected reduction in renal function with nephroureterectomy that could potentially preclude cisplatin-based chemotherapy in an adjuvant setting.

Case 4: A patient undergoes nephroureterectomy and lymphadenectomy for a pT1 high grade (HG) UTUC.

Question 5: Is lymphadenectomy necessary in this situation and if so to what extent?

No prospective data exist to address this question, and retrospective data generally come from small cohorts, due to the low incidence of this disease. However, a retrospective multicenter study of 1,130 patients with pT1-T4 disease who underwent radical nephroureterectomy suggested those staged pT2 and higher have better CSS and disease specific survival with lymphadenectomy (7).

Because it is exceedingly difficult to accurately stage UTUC tumors prior to nephroureterectomy, with a very high rate of understaging by endoscopic biopsy, a regional LND is recommended for all patients undergoing radical nephroureterectomy. The recommended template and number of lymph nodes that defines an adequate dissection remain areas of active study.

KEY POINTS

- The benefit of cytoreductive surgery in metastatic UTUC is not known.

(continued)

(continued)

- Limited retrospective studies suggest there may be some benefit for metastatectomy in certain populations with metastatic urothelial cancer. Chemotherapy should be administered before surgery in these patients.
- Neoadjuvant chemotherapy prior to radical nephroureterectomy should be discussed, with particular focus on patients with high-grade histology or a 3-dimensional lesion on imaging, in patients with preoperative renal function that is adequate to receive cisplatin-based therapy.
- Lymphadenectomy at the time of radical nephroureterectomy is considered standard of care.

REFERENCES

1. Abe T, Kitamura H, Obara W, et al. Outcome of metastatectomy for urothelial carcinoma: a multi-institutional retrospective study in Japan. *J Urol.* 2014;191(4):932-936.
2. Bekku K, Saika T, Kobayashi Y, et al. Could salvage surgery after chemotherapy have clinical impact on cancer survival of patients with metastatic urothelial carcinoma? *Int J Clin Oncol.* 2013;18(1):110-115.
3. Lehmann J, Suttmann H, Albers P, et al. Surgery for metastatic urothelial carcinoma with curative intent: the German experience (AUO AB 30/05). *Eur Urol.* 2009;55(6):1293-1299.
4. Siefker-Radtke AO, Walsh GL, Pisters LL, et al. Is there a role for surgery in the management of metastatic urothelial cancer? The M.D. Anderson experience. *J Urol.* 2004;171(1):145-148.
5. Herr HW. Is metastatectomy for urothelial carcinoma worthwhile? *Eur Urol.* 2009;55(6):1300-1301.
6. Porten S, Siefker-Radtke AO, Xiao L, et al. Neoadjuvant chemotherapy improves survival of patients with upper tract urothelial carcinoma. *Cancer.* 2014;120 (12):1794-1799.
7. Roscigno M, Shariat S, Margulis V, et al. Impact of lymph node dissection on cancer specific survival in patients with upper tract urothelial carcinoma treated with radical nephroureterectomy. *J Urol.* 2009;181(6):2482-2489.

Upper Tract Urothelial Carcinoma Survivorship 23

Spencer Craven and Jennifer Marie Taylor

SURVIVAL

While urothelial carcinoma (UC) is the fourth most common cancer, upper tract urothelial carcinomas (UTUCs) account for only 5% to 10% of UC tumors (1). Compared to bladder tumors, UTUC tends to present at a more advanced stage, with almost 60% already invasive at diagnosis (2). UTUC also has a tendency for multifocality, local recurrence, and metastasis. Recurrence of disease in the bladder, which is not considered metastasis, occurs in 22% to 47% of UTUC patients, while recurrence in the contralateral upper tract occurs in 2% to 6% of patients (3). Prognosis for UTUC depends heavily on stage and grade as well as nodal involvement, lymphovascular invasion, and tumor multifocality. Stage Ta and Tis tumors have 5-year survival rates approaching 100%, while 5-year survival rate for stage T3 tumors does not exceed 50% (4).

FOLLOW-UP

Given the poor prognosis for many patients as well as the high rates of recurrence, continued counseling and follow-up after initial diagnosis and treatment are key. All patients should be counseled to quit smoking, as this is a risk factor for all UCs. Patients who have undergone radical nephroureterectomy (RNU) must be counseled on the risks of having only a single functioning renal unit. Studies have shown an association between chronic kidney disease and cardiovascular morbidity and mortality after nephrectomy for renal tumors, which can be extrapolated to RNU patients. The estimated glomerular filtration rate (eGFR) has also been shown to be significantly diminished after RNU, particularly in the elderly (5).

Regular surveillance is necessary in all UTUC patients in order to detect local recurrence, metachronous bladder tumors, and distant metastases. The follow-up for these patients is frequent, expensive, and invasive, adding considerable morbidity to the disease. Both the National Comprehensive Cancer Network (NCCN) and the European Association of Urology (EAU) provide guidelines for surveillance of UTUC. The NCCN recommends uniform follow-up for all stages and treatment modalities including cystoscopy every 3 months for 1 year and then at increasing intervals after that. Imaging of the upper tracts is also recommended at 3 to 12 month intervals (6). The EAU breaks their recommendations down based on treatment modality and tumor characteristics. Following RNU, patients with noninvasive tumors should have cystoscopy and urine cytology at 3 months and then yearly thereafter. Patients with invasive tumors should have an additional CT urogram (CTU) every 6 months over 2 years and then yearly. Patients managed conservatively should receive cytology and CTU at 3 and 6 months followed by yearly exams. Cystoscopy, ureteroscopy, and cytology are recommended at 3 and 6 months, then every 6 months over 2 years, and then yearly thereafter. All conservatively managed patients should be followed for at least 5 years (2). The frequency of surveillance visits speaks to the need for continued comanagement between Urology and Medical Oncology in most cases.

Probabilities of recurrence, metastasis, and death evolve over time and decrease with increased survivorship. This is known as conditional survival (7). For all UTUC patients, 5-year survival increased from 62.6% at the time of treatment to 71.6% after 5 years. This effect is even more pronounced in patients with adverse pathologic features. Patents with pT3-4 disease increased from 39% at the time of treatment to 65% after 5 years. These estimates provide a dynamic view of cancer survivorship for both patients and physicians that can aid in patient counseling and surveillance planning.

> **KEY POINTS**
>
> - Prognostic factors include stage and grade as well as nodal involvement, lymphovascular invasion, and tumor multifocality.
> - UTUC is associated with frequent local recurrence, metachronous bladder tumors, and distant metastases.
> - General health counseling including smoking cessation and renal precautions are encouraged.
> - Screening for recurrence depends on tumor stage/grade and treatment modality and is frequent, expensive, and invasive.
> - Survival rates are based on prognostic factors but have been shown to increase with increasing survivorship (conditional survival).

REFERENCES

1. Munoz JJ, Ellison LM. Upper tract urothelial neoplasms: incidence and survival during the last 2 decades. *J Urol.* 2000;164(5):1523-1525.
2. Rouprêt M, Babjuk M, Böhle A, et al. Guidelines on urothelial carcinoma of the upper urinary tract. *Eur Assoc Urol.* 2015. http://uroweb.org/wp-content/uploads/06-UTUC_druk_LR.pdf. Accessed December 22, 2016.
3. Novara G, De Marco V, Dalpiaz O, et al. Independent predictors of contralateral metachronous upper urinary tract transitional cell carcinoma after nephroureterectomy: multi-institutional dataset from three European centers. *Int J Urol.* 2009;16(2):187-191.
4. Leow JJ, Orsola A, Chang SL, et al. A contemporary review of management and prognostic factors of upper tract urothelial carcinoma. *Cancer Treat Rev.* 2015;41:310-319.
5. Remzi M, Shariat S, Huebner W, et al. Upper urinary tract urothelial carcinoma: what have we learned in the last 4 years? *Ther Adv Urol.* 2011;3(2):69-80.
6. Abbot JE, Cicic A, DiMatteo D, et al. Contemporary management and trends in the treatment of upper tract urothelial carcinoma. *World J Nephrol Urol.* 2015;4(2):189-200.
7. Ploussard G, Xylinas E, Lotan Y, et al. Conditional survival after radical nephroureterectomy for upper tract carcinoma. *Eur Urol.* 2015;67(4):803-812.

BLADDER CANCER

Urothelial Cancer of the Bladder: Treatment of Early Stage Disease

24

Carli Calderone and Jennifer Marie Taylor

INTRODUCTION

Urothelial cancer can arise in the renal pelvis, ureter, bladder, or urethra. This chapter focuses on urothelial cancer of the bladder.

HISTOLOGIC TYPES

Urothelial Carcinoma

By far, the most common histologic type of bladder cancer arises from the urothelium, accounting for greater than 90% of bladder tumors (1). This will be the type predominately discussed in this chapter. Urothelial carcinoma (UC) was formerly known as transitional cell carcinoma (TCC) and is sometimes still referred to as such.

Variants of UC

Up to 25% of UC can demonstrate mixed histological features, many of which portend a worse prognosis (2). These variants include micropapillary, plasmacytoid, nested, sarcomatoid, microcystic, squamous, and adenocarcinoma. In addition to their association with more invasive disease, they also may predict poor response to certain treatments and are an important consideration in treatment decisions.

Non-urothelial Cancers of the Bladder

Squamous cell carcinoma (SCC) accounts for 1% to 2% of bladder tumors and is often invasive at the time of diagnosis. It is associated with chronic inflammation, such as that from long-term indwelling catheters or schistosomiasis infection. In areas where schistosomiasis is endemic, squamous cell cancer is the most common bladder malignancy (3), although rates of UC are a rising proportion given increasing tobacco use in those regions. Likewise, adenocarcinoma contributes to 1% of bladder tumors and is often located at the urachus, where there may be a remnant of nonurothelial epithelium. Small cell carcinoma can also occur in the bladder less than 1% of the time. These tumors tend to grow quickly, metastasize early, and are treated primarily with chemotherapy. Sarcoma arising from bladder muscle is very rare, but may also present as a bladder tumor.

CLASSIFICATION OF BLADDER NEOPLASMS

Grade

The current classification according to the 2004 World Health Organization (WHO) system designates four categories. Urothelial papillomas are completely benign lesions. The term papillary urothelial neoplasm of low malignant potential (PUNLMP) is used to describe premalignant lesions, which exhibit much less aggressive behavior than even the most low-risk UC (4). UC, which will be discussed here, are classified as low grade or high grade.

While no longer in use, occasionally one may come across the terminology used in the 1973 guidelines, especially in prognostic tools. In this former 3-tier system, which assigned from grade 1 to 3, all G1 (well-differentiated) and most G2 (moderately-differentiated) tumors correlate to a 2004 WHO low-grade tumor, while some G2 and all G3 (poorly-differentiated) tumors are considered high grade.

Stage

Bladder tumors are broadly categorized according to depth of bladder wall invasion into nonmuscle-invasive bladder cancer

(NMIBC) and muscle-invasive bladder cancer (MIBC). These two groups generally differentiate bladder cancer based on aggressiveness, risk of metastasis, and treatment options.

The American Joint Committee on Cancer (AJCC) tumor, node, metastasis (TNM) staging system (Table 24.1) is the most widely used system, and can be assigned for both clinical and pathologic stage. Clinical stage is obtained from

Table 24.1 TNM Staging of Bladder Cancer	
Stage	Definition
Ta	Noninvasive, papillary tumor
Tis	Non-invasive, flat (CIS)
T1	Invading lamina propria (subepithelial connective tissue)
T2	Invading muscularis propria pT2a: invades superficial muscularis propria (inner half) pT2b: invades deep muscularis propria (outer half)
T3*	Invading perivesical soft tissue pT3a: microscopically pT3b: macroscopically (extravesical mass)
T4*	Extravesical tumor directly invading into adjacent organ(s) T4a: prostatic stroma, uterus, vagina T4b: pelvic wall, abdominal wall
Nx	Nodal status cannot be determined
N0	No radiographic (or pathologic) evidence of lymph node metastasis
N1	Single positive lymph node in true pelvis
N2	Multiple positive lymph nodes in true pelvis
N3	Lymph node metastasis to common iliac station
Mx	Distant metastasis cannot be determined
M0	No evidence of distant metastasis
M1	Distant metastasis M1a: limited to lymph nodes beyond the common iliacs M1b: non–lymph node distant metastasis

CIS, carcinoma in situ; TNM, tumor, node, metastasis.

Source: Adapted from Ref. (5) American Joint Committee on Cancer. Urinary Bladder. In: Amin MB, Edge SB, Greene FL, et al., eds. *AJCC Cancer Staging Manual,* 8th ed. Chicago, IL: Springer; 2017:757–765.

*Clinical stage T3 or T4 is derived from imaging or exam under anesthesia with palpable or fixed mass

information gathered from transurethral resection of bladder tumor (TURBT), physical exam, and imaging. Pathologic stage is based on operative findings at time of cystectomy. It is generally agreed that a biopsy specimen from TURBT is not substantial enough to constitute pathologic staging, and therefore most NMIBC are classified by their clinical stage (4). Under this system, NMIBC includes stages Ta, T1, and Tis.

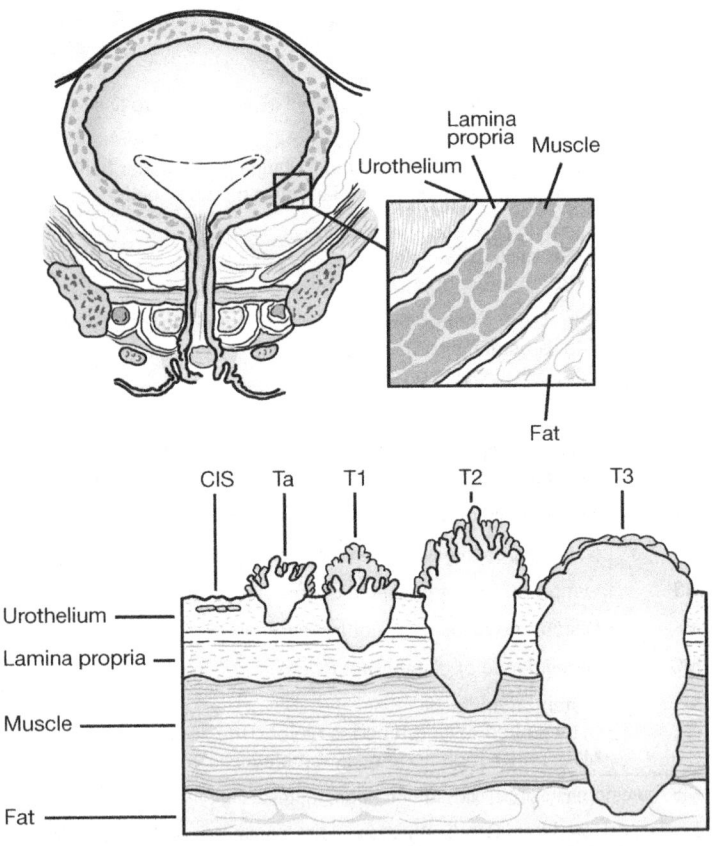

Figure 24.1 Staging.

Source: Adapted from *Bladder Cancer Basics 2nd Edition* with permission from the Bladder Cancer Advocacy Network (BCAN), Bethesda, MD.

Ta: Papillary tumors which are limited to the mucosa are classified as Ta, and describe 70% to 75% of NMIBC at time of diagnosis. Furthermore, the majority of Ta lesions are low grade, with an average of only 6.9% of Ta tumors being high grade (6). The recurrence rates are high, as much as 60% within 5 years; however, the rate of progression to MIBC is rare.

T1: Papillary tumors, which invade the lamina propria, comprise 25% of NMIBC at time of diagnosis (1). Resection by TURBT must include muscle in the specimen for accurate determination of muscle involvement. T1 tumors carry a higher risk of progression to MIBC. However, the overall prognosis is still very good. The presence of lymphovascular invasion has been demonstrated to be a poor prognostic indicator for T1 tumors.

CIS: Carcinoma in situ tumors are flat and confined to the mucosa. They are by definition always high grade, and left untreated, an average of 54% of patients with CIS will progress to MIBC (7). Treatment of CIS can be more challenging to treat and varies considerably from papillary disease, and therefore is often discussed separately.

CIS is further classified into primary, secondary, or concurrent, based on whether the CIS tumor was detected by itself, as a recurrence after prior papillary NMIBC, or concomitantly with papillary disease. Most are concurrent with other high-grade lesions, with only 3% to 5% occurring as isolated CIS.

RISK STRATIFICATION

NMIBC represents a widely heterogeneous group of cancers with highly variable natural histories. Risk stratification is essential to guide management of these patients. In 2016, the American Urological Association (AUA) updated the risk categories for NMIBC, as summarized in Table 24.2 (7). Patients can evolve from one risk group to another as the disease recurs or progresses. This AUA risk stratification is very similar to the system adopted by the European Association of Urology, which has been utilized in research and prediction models. These risk strata correlate with risk of recurrence and progression and align with different choices in the treatment algorithm.

Table 24.2 AUA Risk Stratification for Nonmuscle Invasive Bladder Cancer

Low risk	Intermediate risk	High risk
LG solitary Ta ≤ 3 cm	Recurrence within 1 year, LG Ta	HG T1
PUNLMP	Solitary LG Ta >3 cm	Any recurrent, HG Ta
	LG Ta, multifocal	HG Ta, >3 cm (or multifocal)
	HG Ta, ≤ 3 cm	Any CIS
	LG T1	Any BCG failure in HG patient
		Any variant histology
		Any LVI
		Any HG prostatic urethral involvement

AUA, American Urological Association; CIS, carcinoma in situ; HG, high grade; LG, low grade; LVI, lymphovascular invasion; PUNLMP, papillary urothelial neoplasm of low malignant potential.

CLINICAL PRESENTATION

Risk Factors

Tobacco exposure, both first-hand and second-hand, carries the greatest exposure-related risk for development of bladder cancer. Other occupational and environmental exposures which have been linked to bladder cancer include aromatic amines (e.g., benzenes), aniline dyes, trichloroethylene pesticides, and arsenic. Treatments used for other malignancies, including cyclophosphamide and ionizing pelvic radiation, also may predispose to secondary bladder malignancy. Familial or inherited bladder cancers are rare, but Lynch syndrome is the most common genetic syndrome associated with both upper urinary tract and bladder malignancy.

Despite similar exposure-related risks, UC of the bladder is significantly more prevalent than UC in the upper urothelial tract, due to the cumulative duration of exposure of the urothelium to carcinogens in the urine. This also explains in part the higher incidence of bladder cancer in men relative to women, despite equal rates of tobacco use, due to chronic incomplete bladder emptying associated with age-related prostate enlargement.

Signs and Symptoms

The most common presenting sign of NMIBC is hematuria, either grossly visible to the patient or found incidentally as microscopic hematuria on urinalysis. Gross hematuria is more ominous, with up to 20% of patients demonstrating a urologic malignancy (8). However, even a single episode of unexplained microhematuria necessitates a full work up, including cystoscopy and upper tract imaging, as around 3.3% of these unselected patients may be found to have a urologic malignancy (9).

CIS in particular can cause irritative voiding symptoms, such as frequency, urgency, and dysuria (7). Physical exam is usually normal. Very rarely, NMIBC can lead to obstruction and hydronephrosis, which may present with flank pain or a palpable mass. If hydronephrosis is present from obstruction at the uretero-vesical junction, it is likely to be a more invasive stage.

DIAGNOSTIC WORKUP

Urine Studies

Urine cytology is commonly used as an adjunct to cystoscopy as part of a complete bladder cancer work up. It is more helpful in detecting high grade (HG) tumor cells, where sensitivity has been shown to be 84%, compared to 16% for low grade (LG) tumors (10). Urine cytology is an essential part of diagnosis of CIS and is very specific, although sensitivity varies from 28% to 100%.

Efforts continue to identify urine markers to use as a non-invasive alternative for bladder cancer screening or follow up. At the present time, no marker has demonstrated a high enough sensitivity to replace office cystoscopy. However, when used as adjuncts, some markers have shown promise in providing useful diagnostic information. Once a diagnosis is made, genetic markers have been shown to assist in giving prognostic information, such as recurrence, progression, and even response to therapy.

Cystoscopy

An office-based procedure is typically done for evaluation. Surgical resection by TURBT is necessary for complete diagnostic information and is therapeutic for most cases. Adjuncts to white light cystoscopy, such as narrow band imaging (NBI) and blue light cystoscopy, can improve detection of tumors or lesions and reduce rates of recurrence.

Papillary tumors will be easily visualized and appear grossly as clusters of papillary stalks with a fibrovascular core (see Figure 24.2). Note should be taken endoscopically of tumor appearance (e.g., papillary, nodular, sessile, flat, necrotic), size, location, and number. CIS is more difficult to detect and may appear erythematous or inflamed. A positive urine cytology with a normal-appearing bladder mucosa should raise suspicion for presence of CIS or disease arising in nonbladder urothelium.

Imaging

A CT urogram (CTU), which includes a delayed phase allowing contrast to opacify the urinary tract, provides the most diagnostic information about the upper urothelial tracts. This is especially important in patients that are at high risk for upper tract urinary carcinoma, including patients with multiple tumors or tumors of the trigone (11). Papillary tumors usually appear as filling defects (see Figure 24.3), and obstructing tumors may cause hydroureter and hydronephrosis. CTU also images the regional and retroperitoneal lymph nodes, as well as surrounding structures, and can give information about local and distant extent of disease. Ultrasound, although not used routinely in the assessment of bladder tumors, can be a useful tool when upper tract obstruction is suspected and can be utilized when CT is not feasible or for surveillance of lower-risk patients after initial diagnosis.

24. UROTHELIAL CANCER OF THE BLADDER 165

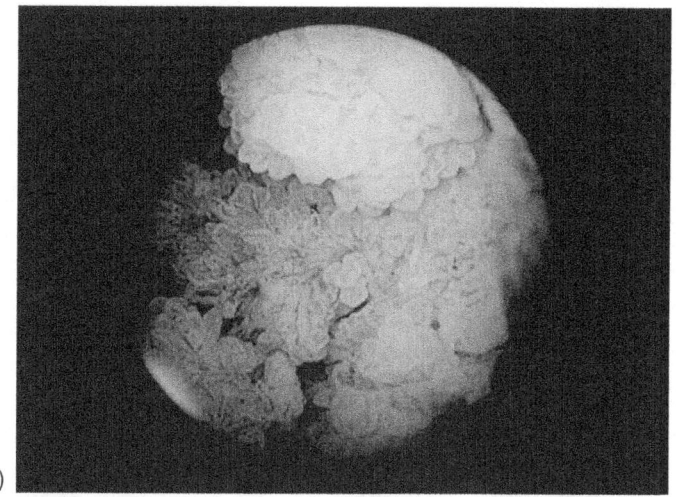

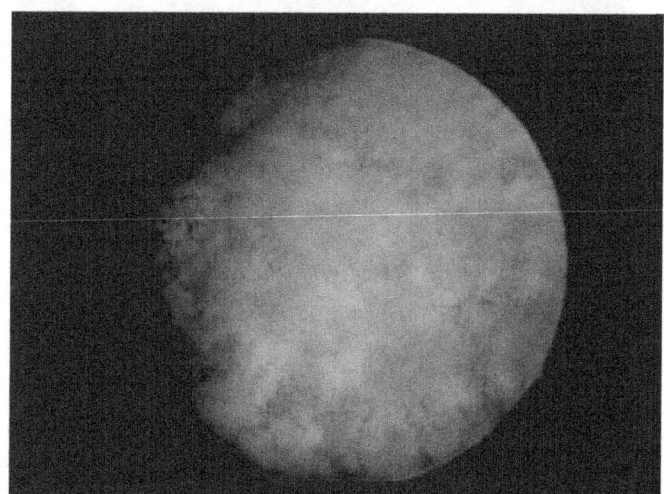

Figure 24.2 Cystoscopy images of (A) papillary bladder tumor and (B) CIS.

CIS, carcinoma in situ.

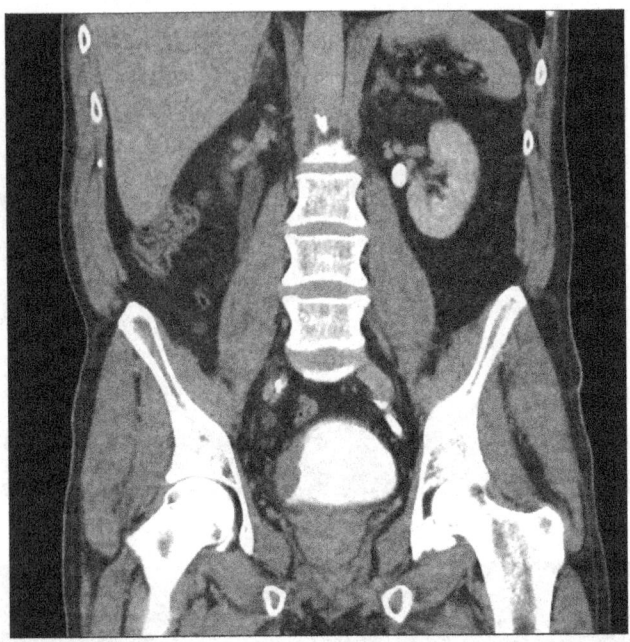

Figure 24.3 Filling defect as seen on CTU suggestive of bladder mass.

CTU, CT urogram.

Visualization Methods

To address the limitations of white light cystoscopy with occult papillary tumors and CIS, improved methods of visualization have been developed. Photodynamic diagnosis (PDD) takes advantage of the fact that photoactive porphyrins accumulate preferentially in neoplastic tissue, which fluoresce pink with exposure to blue light (see Figure 24.4). Multiple studies have demonstrated that PDD increases the detection of tumors and leads to more complete resection (12,13). An optical imaging agent (Hexaminolevulinate HCl, Cysview®, in United States) is instilled in the bladder at least one hour prior to surgery and the cystoscopy camera and image processing unit can alternate between white and blue light.

Similarly, Narrow Band Imaging (NBI) enhances visualization through the use of a light emitted at two specific wavelengths,

24. UROTHELIAL CANCER OF THE BLADDER 167

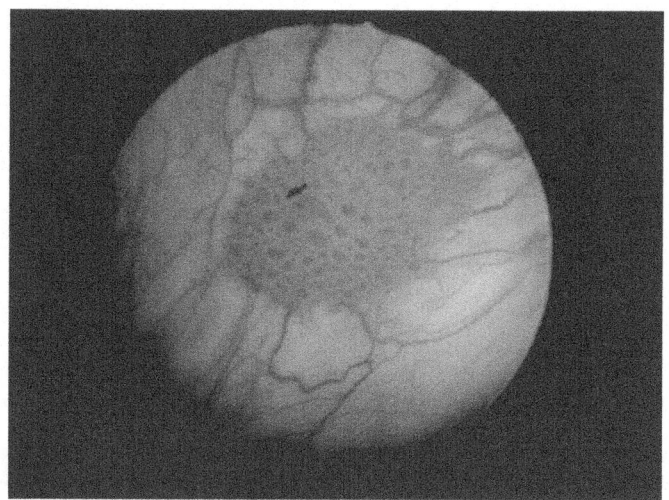

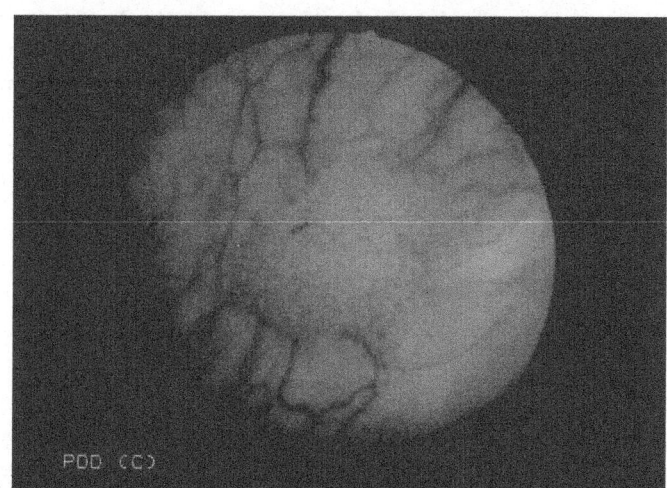

Figure 24.4 Tumor as visualized under (A) white light and (B) blue light.

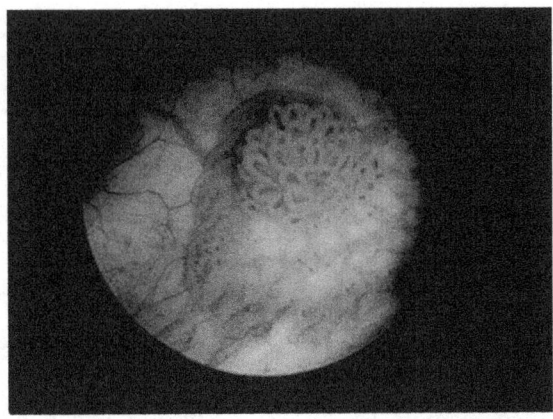

Figure 24.5 Papillary tumor as seen with NBI.

NBI, narrow band imaging.

which are strongly absorbed by hemoglobin and enhance the visualization of capillaries (see Figure 24.5) (14). This technology can be visualized with an NBI camera and processing unit and does not require instillation of an imaging agent. NBI use in conjunction with standard white light has been shown to improve tumor detection and resection, but has yet to demonstrate an improvement in recurrence or progression.

MANAGEMENT

Transurethral Resection of Bladder Tumor

TURBT is the mainstay of the diagnosis of NMIBC. TURBT is best performed in an operating room, where an exam under general anesthesia can be performed to determine clinical stage. All visible tumors should be resected at first TURBT, which is both diagnostic and therapeutic. A good resection specimen should include detrusor muscle to achieve the most accurate staging as well as to minimize the chance of local recurrence (15).

Random or targeted bladder biopsies are sometimes necessary in order to diagnose CIS. Biopsy of prostatic urethra may also be indicated. Tumors at high risk for urethral involvement include CIS, multiple tumors, and tumors located in the trigone or bladder neck.

Repeat Resection

Understaging on initial resection is relatively common and does not necessarily reflect a poor quality resection. Repeat or restaging TURBT has been shown to upstage the initial tumor pathology in 21% of specimens (16). Therefore, the AUA 2016 guidelines recommend a repeat TUR in all patients with T1 tumors and most patients with Ta tumors to assess for muscle invasion, regardless of status of muscle in the initial resection (7). Furthermore, repeat resection has been associated with lower recurrence rates after Bacillus Calmette-Guérin (BCG) (17). Persistent T1 disease on repeat resection carries a higher risk prognosis and may prompt discussion of early cystectomy in select patients.

Intravesical Therapies

Perioperative Instillation

A single, immediate postoperative instillation of intravesical chemotherapy has been found to decrease recurrence of low-risk tumors compared to TURBT alone. One meta-analysis of over 2,000 patients with low- and moderate-risk tumors found that the recurrence rate in those who received intravesical chemotherapy was reduced by 14% when compared to patients who received TURBT alone (18). There was no benefit to patients with high-risk tumors.

Mitomycin C (MMC), epirubicin, and pirarubicin are all effective, with none being shown to be superior to the others. Although none is Food and Drug Administration (FDA) approved, MMC is most commonly used in the United States.

Adjuvant Therapies

Additional adjuvant intravesicular instillations may be indicated for patients with AUA risk groups of intermediate-risk and high-risk tumors. These are broadly grouped into cytotoxic agents and one immunomodulatory agent.

MMC is an alkylating agent, which has been shown to decrease tumor recurrence risk by 38% (7). It is given in weekly instillations for 6 to 8 weeks followed by monthly instillations for up to a year, at a dose of 20 to 60 mg per instillation. Efficacy can be optimized by placing patients NPO for 8 hours prior to instillation, assuring an empty bladder, alkalinizing urine with oral sodium bicarbonate, and concentrating the dose of MMC (19). As a full course agent, it is inferior to BCG in preventing tumor progression and is not considered first line for high-grade disease.

Several other agents including thiotepa, doxorubicin, and epirubicin, which are not used commonly in current practice, continue to be studied in clinical trials.

Valrubicin was approved by the FDA in 2009 for treatment of BCG-unresponsive CIS. **Gemcitabine** has also been shown to have modest effect in the BCG-unresponsive NMIBC patient population. Both of these agents are considered salvage therapy in patients who cannot undergo or refuse cystectomy.

Immunotherapy

BCG is the original immunotherapy developed for bladder cancer, approved in 1998, and is the first-line treatment for adjuvant intravesical treatment of high grade NMIBC and CIS (7). Standard induction therapy is given weekly for 6 weeks, starting 2 to 4 weeks after a primary tumor resection. Maintenance therapy has been shown to further reduce recurrence and progression (20) over induction therapy alone, and is given in 3-week courses at intervals every 3 to 6 months consistent with the original Southwest Oncology Group study. According to 2016 AUA guidelines risk groups, maintenance is recommended up to 1 year in intermediate-risk and up to 3 years in high-risk patients. In patients who have poor tolerance of full-dose BCG, reduced-dose therapy is an alternative to the cessation of therapy.

In the treatment of CIS, BCG has been demonstrated to produce a complete response in up to 84% of patients (6), with approximately 50% of patients remaining disease-free for a median of 4 years. After 10 years, up to 30% remain disease-free. Of those who recur, the vast majority will do so within 5 years. Multiple meta-analyses have been performed comparing BCG to chemotherapy for CIS and papillary NMIBC, and all but one have demonstrated that BCG reduces recurrence and progression. However, a survival benefit has not been demonstrated.

Serious complications occur in less than 5% of patients and most are easily managed (21). Systemic BCG infection is quite rare but may require systemic antituberculous therapy.

There is a relative contraindication to the use of BCG in immunocompromised patients; however, retrospective studies have shown no increased toxicity in these patients, with similar efficacy (22). Furthermore, maintenance therapy is not associated with a higher toxicity than induction therapy alone.

BCG-Unresponsive Disease

The term BCG failure is ambiguous and a 2015 consensus statement (23) highlighted the confusion in the multiple terms for failure or intolerance of BCG treatment. The term "BCG-unresponsive" has been established to create a consistent definition, particularly for eligibility in clinical trials. A patient with BCG-unresponsive disease has recurrent or progressive disease after induction BCG plus at least one course of repeat induction or maintenance therapy. This entity is defined as recurrent or progressive disease after induction BCG plus at least one course of repeat induction or maintenance therapy. Determining persistent CIS can take up to 6 months after therapy, as tumoricidal activity persists after the cessation of therapy.

How to Treat Failure/Intolerance of BCG

Patients who are resistant to their first induction course of BCG or who recur after an initial complete response of at least 12 months should consider a second induction course, as there is a 30% to 50% response with re-treatment (24). However, there is an increased risk of progression. Therefore, high-risk patients who experience early recurrence, multiple recurrences, or disease progression should consider immediate cystectomy. Further courses of BCG beyond two are not recommended, as they portend an 80% failure rate, causing an avoidable delay in treatment.

In those patients who cannot tolerate surgery or refuse cystectomy, salvage intravesical therapies are options and remain active spaces for therapeutic investigation. Valrubicin is the only FDA approved intravesicular therapy to treat such patients with CIS only, and a delay in cystectomy of 3 months to assess efficacy of valrubicin does not appear to increase the risk of progression (25). Gemcitabine has been used for salvage cases, with a moderate response rate (26).

There are no combinations that have been studied to date which have been able to demonstrate a clear benefit over monotherapy with BCG. Interferon when combined as a mixture with BCG was not found to have any additional efficacy in preventing recurrence over BCG alone (27). It demonstrated similar toxicity as well and therefore is not advantageous over BCG monotherapy.

Additional ongoing studies are testing the efficacy of treatment with oncolytic viral therapy, checkpoint inhibitors, IL-2 derivatives, and other agents in this challenging disease setting.

CYSTECTOMY

There is a role for radical cystectomy (RC) in some high-risk patients with NMIBC. Clinical understaging is a real occurrence, with up to 50% of patients with HG NMIBC (<cT1) clinically actually found to have MIBC (>pT2) at cystectomy. One study found that in patients with cT1 + CIS disease who underwent RC, clinical staging was only accurate in 66% of patients, with 27% being upstaged by cystectomy pathology and 12% with positive nodal disease (28). To this end, the AUA guidelines list cystectomy as the first option for refractory disease after initial intravesical therapy.

In addition to tumors which are high-risk, tumors which cannot be reasonably controlled via TURBT should also be considered for cystectomy or partial cystectomy. This may include LG or HG tumors that are bulky or otherwise inaccessible endoscopically, for example due to urethral stricture or bladder diverticulum. Partial cystectomy can allow for more accurate pathologic staging with excision of the specimen and lymph node dissection. The majority of patients can have durable disease-specific survival with an intact, functioning bladder (29).

In conclusion, NMIBC is a complex entity which is not "one-size-fits-all." The majority of cases carry higher risk of recurrence than of progression or metastasis. It carries a high burden of cost and potential morbidity from long-term and multiple interventions, and outcomes can be affected by patient adherence.

> **KEY POINTS**
>
> - Approximately 80% of urothelial bladder cancers are nonmuscle invasive at the time of diagnosis.
> - Risk stratification of NMIBC at time of diagnosis should guide treatment recommendations and surveillance schedules.
> - Intravesical therapy, both as immediate perioperative administration and adjuvant therapy can reduce a patient's risk of recurrence and progression.
> - Increasing grade, stage, or number of tumors correlates with increasing risk of progression.

REFERENCES

1. Fleshner NE, Herr HW, Stewart AK, et al. The National Cancer Data Base report on bladder carcinoma. The American College of Surgeons Commission on Cancer and the American Cancer Society. *Cancer.* 1996;78(7):1505-1513.
2. Wasco MJ, Daignault S, Zhang Y, et al. Urothelial carcinoma with divergent histologic differentiation (mixed histologic features) predicts the presence of locally advanced bladder cancer when detected at transurethral resection. *Urology.* 2007;70(1):69-74.
3. Mostafa MH, Sheweita SA, O'Connor PJ. Relationship between schistosomiasis and bladder cancer. *Clin Microbiol Rev.* 1999;12(1):97-111.
4. Pavone-Macaluso M, Lopez-Beltran A, Aragona F, et al. The pathology of bladder cancer; an update on selected issues. *BJU Int* 2006;98(6):1161-1165.
5. American Joint Committee on Cancer. Urinary bladder. In: Amin MB, Edge SB, Greene FL, et al., eds. *AJCC Cancer Staging Manual,* 8th ed. Chicago, IL: Springer; 2017:757-765.
6. Sylvester RJ, van der Meijden A, Witjes JA, et al. High-grade Ta urothelial carcinoma and carcinoma in situ of the bladder. *Urology.* 2005;66(6):90-107.
7. Chang SS, Boorjian SA, Chou R, et al. Diagnosis and treatment of non-muscle invasive bladder cancer: AUA/SUO Guideline. *J Urol.* 2016;196(4):1021-1029.
8. Khadra MH, Pickard RS, Charlton M, et al. A prospective analysis of 1,930 patients with hematuria to evaluate current diagnostic practice. *J Urol.* 2000;163(2):524-527.

9. Davis R, Jones JS, Barocas DA, et al. Diagnosis, evaluation and follow-up of asymptomatic microhematuria (AMH) in adults: AUA guideline. *J Urol.* 2012;188(6 Suppl):2473-2481.
10. Yafi FA, Brimo F, Steinberg J, et al. Prospective analysis of sensitivity and specificity of urinary cytology and other urinary biomarkers for bladder cancer. *Urol Oncol.* 2015;33(2):66.e25-66.e31.
11. Palou J, Rodríguez-Rubio F, Huguet J, et al. Multivariate analysis of clinical parameters of synchronous primary superficial bladder cancer and upper urinary tract tumor. *J Urol.* 2005;174(3):859-861.
12. Stenzl A, Penkoff H, Dajc-Sommerer E, et al. Detection and clinical outcome of urinary bladder cancer with 5-aminolevulinic acid-induced fluorescence cystoscopy. *Cancer.* 2010;117(5):938-947.
13. Gkritsios P, Hatzimouratidis K, Kazantzidis S, et al. Hexaminolevulinate-guided transurethral resection of non-muscle-invasive bladder cancer does not reduce the recurrence rates after a 2-year follow-up: a prospective randomized trial. *Int Urol Nephrol.* 2013;46(5):927-933.
14. Zheng C, Lv Y, Zhong Q, et al. Narrow band imaging diagnosis of bladder cancer: systematic review and meta-analysis. *BJU Int.* 2012;110(11b):E680-E687.
15. Mariappan P, Zachou A, Grigor KM. Detrusor muscle in the first, apparently complete transurethral resection of bladder tumour specimen is a surrogate marker of resection quality, predicts risk of early recurrence, and is dependent on operator experience. *Eur Urol.* 2010;57(5):843-849.
16. Schwaibold HE, Sivalingam S, May F, et al. The value of a second transurethral resection for T1 bladder cancer. *BJU Int.* 2006;97(6):1199-1201.
17. Herr HW. Restaging transurethral resection of high risk superficial bladder cancer improves the initial response to Bacillus Calmette-Guérin therapy. *J Urol.* 2005;174(6):2134-2137.
18. Sylvester RJ, Oosterlinck W, Holmang S, et al. Systematic review and individual patient data meta-analysis of randomized trials comparing a single immediate instillation of chemotherapy after transurethral resection with transurethral resection alone in patients with stage pTa-pT1 urothelial carcinoma of the bladder: Which patients benefit from the instillation? *Eur Urol.* 2016;69(2):231-244.
19. Au JL, Badalament RA, Wientjes MG, et al. Methods to improve efficacy of intravesical mitomycin C: results of a randomized phase III trial. *J Natl. Cancer Inst.* 2001;93(8):597-604.
20. Han RF, Pan JG. Can intravesical bacillus Calmette-Guérin reduce recurrence in patients with superficial bladder cancer? A meta-analysis of randomized trials. *Urol.* 2006;67(6):1216-1223.

21. Van der Meijden APM, Sylvester RJ, Oosterlinck W, et al. Maintenance Bacillus Calmette-Guérin for Ta T1 bladder tumors is not associated with increased toxicity: Results from a European Organisation for Research and Treatment of Cancer Genito-Urinary Group Phase III Trial. *Eur Urol.* 2003;44(4):429-434.
22. Prabharasuth D, Moses KA, Bernstein M, et al. Management of bladder cancer after renal transplantation. *Urol.* 2013;81(4):813-819.
23. Kamat AM, Flaig TW, Grossman HB, et al. Expert consensus document: consensus statement on best practice management regarding the use of intravesical immunotherapy with BCG for bladder cancer. *Nature Rev Urol.* 2015;12:225-235.
24. Bui TT, Schellhammer PF. Additional Bacillus Calmette-Guérin therapy for recurrent transitional cell carcinoma after an initial complete response. *Urol.* 1997;49(5):687-690.
25. Grossman HB, O'Donnell MA, Cookson MS, et al. Bacillus Calmette-Guérin failures and beyond: contemporary management of non-muscle-invasive bladder cancer. *Rev Urol.* 2008; 10(4):281-289.
26. Skinner EC, Goldman B, Sakr WA, et al. SWOG S0353: phase II trial of intravesical gemcitabine in patients with nonmuscle invasive bladder cancer and recurrence after 2 prior courses of intravesical Bacillus Calmette-Guérin. *J Urol.* 2013;190(4):1200-1204.
27. Bazarbashi S, Soudy H, Abdelsalam M, et al. Co-administration of intravesical Bacillus Calmette-Guérin and interferon alpha-2B as first line in treating superficial transitional cell carcinoma of the urinary bladder. *BJU Int.* 2011;108(7):1115-1118.
28. Bianco FJ Jr, Justa D, Grignon DJ, et al. Management of clinical T1 bladder transitional cell carcinoma by radical cystectomy. *Urol Oncol.* 2004;22(4):290-294.
29. Holzbeierlein JM, Lopez-Corona E, Bochner BH, et al. Partial cystectomy: a contemporary review of the Memorial Sloan-Kettering Cancer Center experience and recommendations for patient selection. *J Urol.* 2004;172(3):878-881.

Management of Invasive Bladder Cancer: Surgery, Chemotherapy, and Radiation Therapy

25

Arun Rai, Thiri Khin, Teresa Gray Hayes, and Jennifer Marie Taylor

INTRODUCTION

Bladder cancer is the most common cancer arising from the urothelial tract, and the ninth most common cancer worldwide. In the United States, it is the fifth most common cancer behind breast, lung, prostate, and colorectal cancer. It accounts for 77,000 new cases each year and 16,000 deaths (1). Urothelial or transitional cell carcinoma comprises 90% of all bladder cancer cases in the United States and Western Europe, of which approximately 25% to 30% of cases are muscle invasive bladder cancer (MIBC).

Despite the utilization of radical cystectomy (RC) for MIBC, the early dissemination of micrometastases frequently results in failure to cure with surgery alone. American Joint Committee on Cancer (AJCC) tumor, node, metastasis (TNM) staging is the definitive staging criteria used for bladder cancer (see Table 24.1) (2).

The recurrence rate after surgery is 20% to 30% in pT1 and pT2 disease and 50% to 90% in pT3 or pT4 (3,4). Clinical understaging has been well documented, and ranges from 31% to 61% (4). Pathologic staging shows extravesical disease (pT3–T4) rates between 25% and 35%, and 5-year survival of patients with MIBC is at best 65%. Approximately 50% of patients will develop metastatic disease within 2 years. Metastatic bladder cancer is aggressive. The efficacy of chemotherapy in metastatic disease has led to the investigation of its use in the perioperative setting with the intent of eradicating micrometastatic disease.

CLINICAL CONSIDERATIONS AND DISEASE PROGRESSION

Of those with muscle invasive disease diagnosed at resection, the majority of patients are diagnosed de novo. Approximately 20% of patients will have progressed from previously diagnosed nonmuscle-invasive disease. The risk of progression is highest within the first 2 years after diagnosis with increasing risk of progression with higher initial stage and grade. As noted in the previous section, T1 tumors have a recurrence rate as high as 50% at 2 years and up to 50% likelihood at 5 years of progression to MIBC. Carcinoma in situ (CIS) is associated with both high rates of recurrence and progression, with the greatest 5-year risk of progression (74%) in a patient with T1 high grade (HG) disease with CIS present (5).

Certain genetic changes have been correlated with earlier incidence of more aggressive, muscle-invasive disease. This includes allelic loss of chromosome 9, loss of Rb1 and p53, and abnormalities in proliferation genes such as *Ki67*. On review of transurethral resection of the bladder tumor (TURBT) pathologic samples, the presence and loss of these genetic markers can help to indicate likelihood of progression to muscle invasive disease. Emerging molecular data from The Cancer Genome Atlas (TCGA) and other characterization studies will provide new insights into the molecular drivers of recurrence and progression and provide avenues to guide treatment.

Pure variant histology tumors other than urothelial bladder cancer are associated with statistically significantly poorer outcomes when compared to primary urothelial carcinoma. However, mixed histology cases, with urothelial and variant histology, occur commonly as the tumors de-differentiate. The incidence of pure squamous cell carcinoma of the bladder is 3% to 7% in the United States, and adenocarcinoma <2%. Other nonurothelial tumors (small cell, carcinosarcoma, lymphoma, neurofibroma, and sarcoma) each occur in less than 1% of bladder cancers in the United States (6).

STAGING CONSIDERATIONS IN BLADDER CANCER

Clinical understaging of T stage, by both resection and physical and radiographic examination, remains a common problem. Up to 40% of patients clinically diagnosed with T1 disease who undergo cystectomy are found to have pathologic T2 disease at surgery. Re-resection of initially diagnosed T1 high-grade disease is required within 2 to 6 weeks to assure appropriate staging. The presence of persistent T1 carcinoma on re-resection is a statistically significant predictor of poor outcome in patients treated with Bacillus Calmette-Guérin (BCG), and an indication for "early" RC. (7) On re-resection, approximately 50% of patients are found to have residual tumor, and 25% of patients will be upstaged from Ta to T1 or from T1 to T2 (7). Certain risk factors increase the likelihood of concomitant or metachronous upper tract urothelial disease. These include high-grade tumor, periureteral location, multiple tumors, bladder CIS, and the presence of vesicoureteral reflux.

On cystoscopy, muscle invasive tumors are often more nodular or sessile in appearance and may have more elements of tissue necrosis (see Figure 25.1). At the time of tumor resection, bimanual exam under anesthesia forms the basis of the TNM clinical T stage, with higher non-organ-confined stage suggested by asymmetric thickening (cT3) or palpable

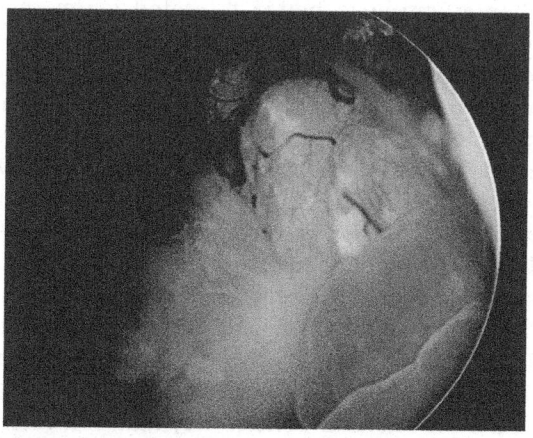

Figure 25.1 Muscle invasive bladder cancer, as seen by cystoscopy.

extension to pelvic sidewall or adjacent organ (cT4). By imaging such as CT urography (CTU), muscle invasive tumors often show focal bladder wall thickening or can cause obstruction with resulting hydronephrosis if located near the ureteral orifice. Perivesical stranding on axial imaging, when obtained prior to transurethral resection, is highly suspicious for microscopic or macroscopic extravesical extension (stage cT3).

For patients diagnosed with MIBC, axial imaging of the abdomen and pelvis is required for staging, for examination of lymph nodes and visceral organs, particularly liver. Chest imaging with chest x-ray is indicated, while chest axial imaging CT may be advised in higher risk patients. A bone scan may be obtained in patients with concerning symptoms.

Indications for RC include resectable muscle invasive disease (clinical stages T2–T4a N0 M0), BCG-unresponsive CIS, high-risk histology with persistent T1 disease on repeat resection, or T1 tumors with associated CIS, lymphovascular invasion (LVI), or variant histology (the latter being a Grade C American Urological Association [AUA] recommendation) (7).

RATIONALE FOR NEOADJUVANT CHEMOTHERAPY

Giving chemotherapy prior to surgery has several advantages. Chemotherapy is better tolerated when the patient has a better performance status than in the postoperative state. Neoadjuvant chemotherapy can downstage the tumor, which may lead to a better surgical outcome. The ability to assess pathologic response to chemotherapy in the surgical specimen can be used for prognostication, and the effectiveness of chemotherapy can help guide the use of later lines of treatment if needed. The major downside of neoadjuvant chemotherapy is the need to rely on clinical stage, which may be inaccurate and can either downstage or upstage the tumor. There is also a concern for morbidity caused by neoadjuvant chemotherapy, which could cause a delay to RC, although recent reports suggest no statistical difference. A lack of predictable data for survival benefit may lead to overtreatment of a portion of patients who otherwise would not need chemotherapy (8–10).

BENEFITS OF NEOADJUVANT CHEMOTHERAPY

A pivotal Southwest Oncology Group (SWOG) 8701/US Intergroup trial compared neoadjuvant MVAC (methotrexate, vinblastine, Adriamycin, cisplatin), followed by RC versus RC alone (11) and found the chemotherapy group to have a median overall survival of 77 months compared to 46 months for those undergoing RC alone. The 5-year overall survival did not reach statistical significance at 57% versus 43% ($P = .06$). Pathological complete response (pCR) rates were 38% versus 15%.

The International Collaboration of Trialists Study is the largest phase 3 randomized prospective trial of neoadjuvant chemotherapy for bladder cancer. This trial enrolled 976 patients and compared neoadjuvant CMV (cisplatin, methotrexate, vinblastine) followed by local therapy versus local therapy alone. The updated report shows a 10-year overall survival of 36% versus 30% for local therapy alone, with a hazard ratio (HR) of 0.84 (12).

The Nordic cystectomy trials I and II compared neoadjuvant chemotherapy with cisplatin and doxorubicin in Nordic I and CMV in Nordic II followed by cystectomy. The trials failed to show an overall survival or cancer specific survival benefit. However, subgroup analysis of the patients with T3 and T4 disease showed an absolute survival benefit of 15% in the patients who received chemotherapy (13). Meta-analysis of 11 prospective trials using neoadjuvant chemotherapy was conducted by the Medical Research Council Clinical Trials unit and reported by the Advanced Bladder Cancer Meta-Analysis Collaboration. It included 3,005 patients and demonstrated a 5% absolute survival benefit with HR 0.86 ($P = .003$) and 9% absolute disease-free survival benefit, HR 0.78 ($P < .0001$) (14).

Across multiple trials, the lowest long-term recurrence and best survival outcomes are seen in patients who achieve pathologic T0 stage after chemotherapy (15,16).

HOW TO CHOOSE NEOADJUVANT CHEMOTHERAPY REGIMENS

There is no evidence of superiority of one chemotherapy regimen over another, since none of the conventional regimens have been compared head-to-head. However, better tolerability and comparable efficacy of gemcitabine and cisplatin (GC) in metastatic disease have led to its adoption for neoadjuvant chemotherapy, and GC has become the most commonly used regimen. Zargar et al. reported retrospective data of comparison of neoadjuvant MVAC, GC, and other regimens in MIBC (9). There was no statistically significant difference in pathological response between MVAC and GC (24.5% vs. 23.9%) or overall survival.

Dose-dense MVAC, which increases the dose intensity of MVAC by administering treatment every 2 weeks along with granulocyte colony-stimulating factor (G-CSF) support, has been studied in metastatic urothelial cancer, but there is no randomized trial evaluating efficacy in the neoadjuvant setting. Two single arm phase 2 studies showed the feasibility of administering three to four cycles of dose-dense MVAC in the neoadjuvant setting, with a pathological complete response rate (pCR) up to 38% (8,11). Given a shortened time to surgery, dose-dense MVAC remains a reasonable alternative and continues to be actively studied in trials.

Multiple phase 2 trials have been conducted to add novel agents such as bevacizumab, lapatinib, and erlotinib to combination cisplatin-based chemotherapy. The addition of bevacizumab led to increased surgical complications. Data for targeted therapy are still at large.

REGIMENS TO USE IN PATIENTS WITH RENAL INSUFFICIENCY

The median age at diagnosis of bladder cancer is 69 years in men and 71 years in women. Comorbidities and functional status are major factors influencing the choices of treatment modality. Renal insufficiency is often encountered in bladder cancer patients due to urinary outflow tract obstruction, advanced age, and/or coexisting medical conditions. In patients with renal insufficiency, there is an unmet need for effective chemotherapy other than the nephrotoxic agent cisplatin. Carboplatin-based neoadjuvant chemotherapy was evaluated in several phase 2 trials, with a pCR rate up to 30% to 40%. Compared to cisplatin, there was more myelosuppression and a higher treatment related mortality. In the therapy of metastatic disease, carboplatin has been shown to be inferior to cisplatin (8,10). Therefore, carboplatin-based chemotherapy is not currently recommended in the neoadjuvant setting. In patients with mild to moderate renal insufficiency who are good surgical candidates, upfront RC is recommended in clinical practice.

ROLE OF SURGERY

RC is critical in the management of local tumor control. Similar to the results found with neoadjuvant chemotherapy, optimizing the likelihood of complete pathologic response in the final tumor specimen has been shown to improve overall survival (3). Resection in men includes prostate, seminal vesicles, distal ureters, pelvic peritoneum, and bladder. For women, the uterus, cervix, ovaries, anterior vagina, distal ureters, pelvic peritoneum, and bladder are removed. During RC, a bilateral pelvic lymph node dissection should be performed, to include lymph nodes in the external iliac, internal iliac, obturator, and common iliac stations. The oncologic efficacy and comparative benefit of minimally invasive (robotic-assisted) cystectomy, relative to open surgery, continues to be studied.

Although neoadjuvant therapy is key to the achievement of a pathologic T0 specimen, some patients can achieve pT0 status from the initial TURBT. On the other hand, restaging with cystoscopy and biopsies cannot always detect occult persistent disease, and RC is required to achieve survival benefit due to the persistence of microscopic disease. Relapse has been demonstrated in up to 64% of patients who maintained their bladders despite apparent complete neoadjuvant response (16). During RC, a bilateral pelvic lymph node dissection should be performed. The oncologic efficacy and comparative benefit of minimally invasive (robotic-assisted) cystectomy, relative to open surgery, continues to be studied. For patients who are not deemed to be cystectomy candidates, trimodal bladder preservation therapy is an option (see section on Bladder Preservation).

SURGICAL CONSIDERATIONS

Perioperative (90-day) mortality rates are 1% to 3% at large centers, but can be significantly higher in community hospitals. Up to 64% of patients, even in high-volume centers of expertise, experience at least one perioperative complication within 90 days, and 13% experience a high-grade (grade 3 or higher) complication (17). Patients older than 70 years have a baseline 3- to 5-fold increase in perioperative mortality even when they are without significant comorbidities (18). In general, patients with significant medical comorbidity are best served by alternative approaches, albeit with potentially less durable benefit. The risk of complications can be minimized by proper patient selection, using objective assessment instruments when possible, and protocols to standardize perioperative management. These include principles known as Enhanced Recovery after Surgery (ERAS), covering elements of physical conditioning, nutrition, fluid management, postoperative diet, and other subjects (see Figure 25.2). The risk of venous thromboembolic events (VTE) is known to be increased in cancer patients undergoing pelvic surgery, and recent data have described

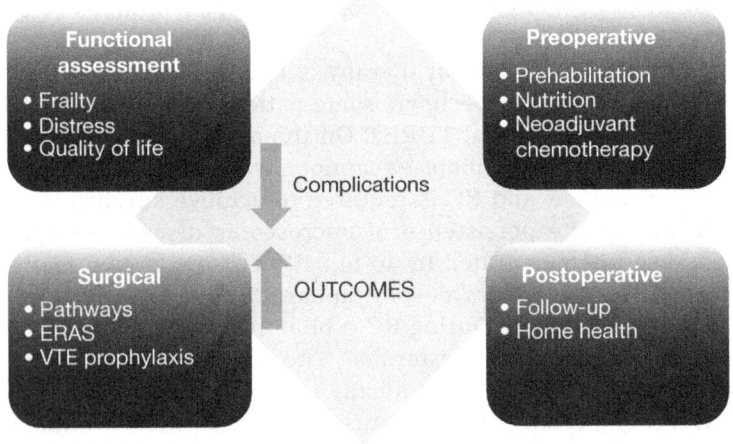

Figure 25.2 Elements of perioperative optimization.

ERAS, enhanced recovery after surgery; VTE, venous thromboembolic event.

much higher rates of VTE in patients receiving platinum-based chemotherapy. Surgeons are increasingly aware of these risks and may incorporate preoperative and extended postoperative VTE prophylaxis to reduce the risk of a potentially fatal complication such as pulmonary embolism.

In the SWOG 8710 trial, negative surgical soft tissue margins and removal of 10 or more lymph nodes were significantly associated with longer survival and decreased local recurrence. Achieving negative soft tissue margins is critical in resection, and positive soft tissue margins carry a significant risk of recurrence and progression (19). Further analysis demonstrated that improved surgical outcomes could be achieved by centralizing the treatment of locally advanced bladder cancer at high-volume institutions with experienced surgeons.

A typical postoperative course generally consists of a 4 to 7 day hospital stay, allowing for recovery of bowel function, along with adequate ambulation and pain control. Patients often take several months to recover their strength and appetites fully, and many benefit from postoperative rehabilitation, either in a facility or at home. Optimal perioperative care incorporates the patient's family members and considers their physical, psychosocial, and functional needs. A multidisciplinary team could include a nutritionist, social worker, psychologist, physical/occupational therapist, and patient navigator, along with the medical and surgical clinicians, and the integration of these varied aspects of care can contribute to better recovery and quality of life.

Intraoperative Frozen Section: The urothelial margin status at the urethral stump is important if orthotopic diversion is considered. Prostatic urethral involvement by urothelial cancer, particularly at the urethral margin of resection, is associated with risk of urethral and pelvic recurrence. In general, tumors involving the bladder neck carry increased risk of urethral involvement and often preclude orthotopic neobladder construction (20).

Urinary Diversion Overview: The type of urinary tract reconstruction is determined after careful preoperative evaluation of the patient's comorbidities and functional status. The types can be broadly classified into incontinent (ileal/colonic segment) or continent diversions (summarized in Table 25.1). All diversions lead to chronic bacteriuria due to persistent bowel flora in the urinary system (21).

Table 25.1 Types of Urinary Diversion

Type of Diversion	Advantages	Disadvantages	Contraindications
Ileal Conduit	Most commonly used, technically simpler, easier management and maintenance for patient	Progressive upper tract deterioration, urinary tract infections (UTIs), stomal/parastomal hernias, stomal stenosis, peristomal skin irritation, ulceration, stomal bleeding (up to 10%), pyelonephritis	Inflammatory bowel disease, bowel malignancy, malabsorption disorders
Continent Cutaneous Diversion Segment of bowel, commonly ileocecal, serves as a reservoir with catheterizable limb on abdominal wall	Improved cosmesis, lifestyle, and independence, decreased risk of reflux	Urolithiasis, stomal stenosis UTIs, longer length of surgery, urinary incontinence, delay until optimal bladder function, requires longer harvested bowel segment	Poor patient dexterity/functional status, hepatic dysfunction, poor renal function
Orthotopic Diversion Consists of an afferent limb that empties into an ileal reservoir anastomosed to native urethra	Cosmesis, lifestyle, and independence	Urolithiasis, UTIs, longer length of surgery, urinary incontinence, delay until optimal bladder function, requires longer harvested bowel segment	Multiple comorbidities and/or poor functional status of patient, poor renal function, history of urethral stricture, positive urethral margin, extensive extravesical disease, pubic bone involvement, plan for postoperative pelvic radiation

25. MANAGEMENT OF INVASIVE BLADDER CANCER 187

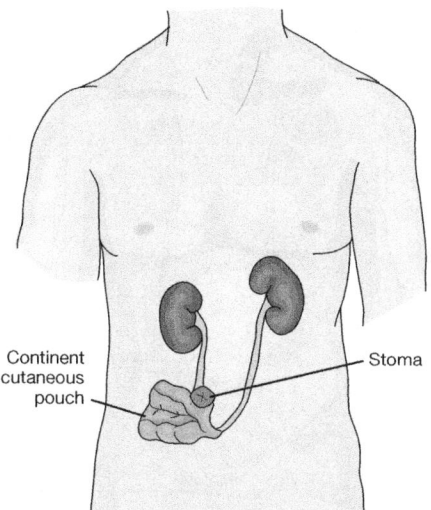

Figure 25.3A A continent cutaneous pouch.

Source: Adapted from *Bladder Cancer Basics 2nd edition* with permission from the Bladder Cancer Advocacy Network (BCAN), Bethesda, MD.

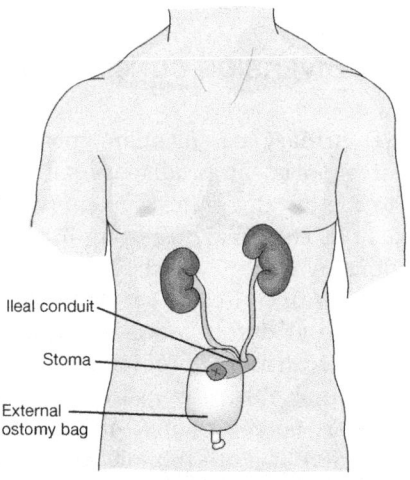

Figure 25.3B Ileal conduit.

Source: Adapted from *Bladder Cancer Basics 2nd edition* with permission from the Bladder Cancer Advocacy Network (BCAN), Bethesda, MD.

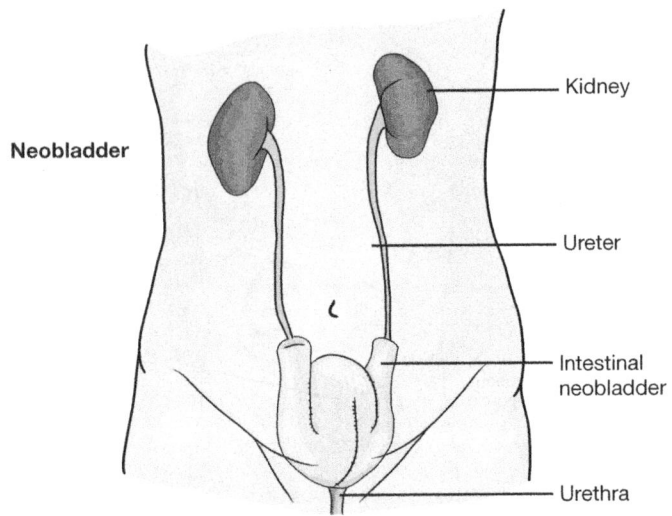

Figure 25.3C Neobladder.

Source: Adapted from *Bladder Cancer Basics 2nd edition* with permission from the Bladder Cancer Advocacy Network (BCAN), Bethesda, MD.

POSTOPERATIVE DIVERSION CONSIDERATIONS

Chronic bacterial urinary colonization, metabolic derangements, and hypercalciuria can predispose patients with intestinal diversion to the development of magnesium ammonium phosphate stones (3). The incidence of urolithiasis in patients with colon conduits is 3% to 5% and 10% to 12% in ileal conduits, and up to 20% with continent cecal reservoirs. Metabolic derangements can occur due to bowel segment absorption of electrolytes in urine. Nutritional problems can result from loss of significant intestinal absorptive surface. In patients with ileal and colonic-derived diversions, vitamin B_{12} malabsorption has been reported. If more than 60 to 100 cm of ileum is resected (increased risk in orthotopic neobladders), the risk of malabsorption of bile acids increases.

Role for Adjuvant Chemotherapy

To date, no prospective comparison between neoadjuvant and adjuvant chemotherapy in muscle-invasive bladder cancer has been carried out. Given the survival benefit with neoadjuvant chemotherapy, treatment before surgery is recommended for eligible patients with MIBC. Patients who undergo RC and are found to have high-risk features, defined as pathologic stage T3 and T4, positive soft tissue margins, and/or positive nodal disease, are offered adjuvant chemotherapy. However, a significant proportion of patients who undergo RC develop complications, which may preclude them from getting additional therapy in a timely fashion.

The benefit of adjuvant chemotherapy is shown in a meta-analysis of nine trials with 945 patients total (22), which showed improvement in overall survival (HR 0.77, 95% confidence interval [CI] 0.59–0.99) and also improvement in disease-free survival (HR 0.66, 95% CI 0.45–0.91). However, this meta-analysis had multiple flaws: all studies had lower accrual than planned and several studies terminated prematurely. The largest and most recent European Organisation for Research and Treatment of Cancer (EORTC) 30994 trial, not included in the meta-analysis, randomized 284 patients to four cycles of adjuvant chemotherapy versus observation, with administration of six cycles of chemotherapy upon relapse (23). This study showed a trend toward improvement in overall survival of 53.6% versus 47.7%, which did not reach statistical significance (HR 0.78, 95% CI 0.56–1.08). More clinical trials are needed to identify the patient population that will benefit the most from neoadjuvant/adjuvant chemotherapy and regimens that minimize the adverse effects of chemotherapy.

Bladder Preservation

RC has long been the standard of care in the management of MIBC. However, due to substantial perioperative morbidity in an older patient population that often has underlying medical comorbidities, bladder preservation techniques have been explored. Though there are no prospective randomized control trials comparing RC to bladder sparing techniques, many clinicians believe bladder-sparing techniques have inferior oncologic outcomes. The major drawback is disease recurrence in the retained bladder, which is estimated to be 50% or more by 3 to 5 years after surgery.

Options for a bladder preservation approach include radical transurethral resection (TUR), partial cystectomy and radiation therapy (RT), and combined chemoradiation. A retrospective study showed TUR had a similar 10-year survival rate compared to RC in muscle invasive cancer that was stage T0 to T1 at the time of TUR restaging (24). For solitary tumors, partial cystectomy is another viable option. A series of 58 highly selected patients reported a 5-year survival rate of 69%, with 74% alive with bladder intact (25). One must be cautioned that such series are done in large-volume centers with very strict selection criteria, very close follow-up, and lifelong cystoscopy. For patients who are not candidates for RC due to comorbidities and those who wish to retain their bladders, optimal candidates for bladder preservation techniques include those with a single tumor less than 5 cm in size, absence of CIS (Tis), clinical T2 or T3a disease, absence of hydronephrosis, and good bladder and renal function.

Role of RT

RT for MIBC is commonly used as a palliative approach to control local symptoms in frail, medically unfit patients. External beam radiation therapy (EBRT) and brachytherapy combined with EBRT are two available options. The local recurrence rate for EBRT when used alone is estimated as high as 70%, and thus this modality alone should not be used in otherwise healthy patients. In patients with a single tumor less than 5 cm, a large European study showed that there was no difference in 5- or 10-year disease-free survival when brachytherapy combined with EBRT was compared to RC (26). The 10-year overall survival was better in the RC group (42% vs. 33% with brachytherapy). Results may have been confounded by a younger patient population in the cystectomy group (26).

Maximal transurethral resection followed by combined chemotherapy and RT, also called trimodal therapy, is an appropriate alternative for patients who are not candidates for radical cystectomy. In patients who are surgical candidates, trimodal therapy is employed frequently outside the United States and in select centers in the United States. When done at centers with experience and with careful post-treatment surveillance, patients can derive similar cancer and quality of life outcomes. Combined chemotherapy with RT has shown superior outcomes in local and regional control and trends toward improvement in survival when compared to RT alone (27). Most commonly used chemotherapy regimens are cisplatin-based, but a 5-fluorouracil and mitomycin combination may be employed in patients with impaired renal function. A Radiation Therapy Oncology Group (RTOG)-pooled analysis of six trials showed a 10-year disease-specific survival of 65% and a 10-year overall survival of 36% (28). One U.S. center with experience treating 465 patients over 25 years (29) has reported steadily improving survival outcomes over time, with an initial complete response rate of 76% and salvage RC performed in 27% for either incomplete response or recurrence. Long-term follow-up among complete responders shows 5- and 10-year disease-specific survival rates of 66% and 59%, with good patient-reported quality of life outcomes (30).

SURVEILLANCE

Careful surveillance should be undertaken for all bladder cancer patients, consisting of surveillance cystoscopy in patients with intact bladder; upper tract monitoring with CT urogram, retrograde pyelograms, or renal ultrasound; and urinary cytology. The schedule and intensity of surveillance depends on risk stratification and recurrence history (31). Following cystectomy, interval abdominal imaging with CT or MRI is warranted to monitor for pelvic or visceral metastatic recurrence. Cytology samples should include a diversion specimen biannually and urethral wash annually if ileal conduit diversion was performed.

KEY POINTS

- The gold standard of care for operable MIBC is neoadjuvant chemotherapy followed by RC.
- In general, organ-confined muscle-invasive disease is the primary indication for RC. However, persistent T1 HG disease, BCG-refractory CIS, or unresectable non-muscle invasive disease are indications for early RC.
- RC involves the removal of prostate, seminal vesicles, distal ureters, pelvic peritoneum, and bladder in males; and uterus, cervix, ovaries, anterior vagina, distal ureters, pelvic peritoneum, and bladder in females.
- An extended pelvic lymphadenectomy is associated with improved surgical and survival outcomes.
- The type of urinary diversion a patient receives postcystectomy depends on comorbidity and functional status. Ileal conduit is the easiest to manage, while orthotopic neobladders offer improved cosmesis. All diversion approaches are associated with an increased risk for urolithiasis, metabolic derangements, and gastrointestinal tract physiological alterations.
- Neoadjuvant chemotherapy with cisplatin-based chemotherapy has shown overall survival benefit in patients with operable MIBC. Patients with poor glomerular filtration rate (GFR) or who cannot tolerate cisplatin should proceed directly to surgery.
- Despite the lack of definitive evidence favoring adjuvant chemotherapy, most clinicians offer postoperative chemotherapy to patients with high-risk pathologic features.
- The efficacy of novel agents, targeted therapy, and immunotherapy in the neoadjuvant setting remains to be determined.

REFERENCES

1. Siegel RL, Miller KD, Jemal A. Cancer statistics, 2016. *CA Cancer J Clin.* January/February 2016;66(1):7-30.
2. American Joint Committee on Cancer. Urinary bladder. In: Amin MB, Edge SB, Greene FL, et al., eds. *AJCC Cancer Staging Manual,* 8th ed. Chicago, IL: Springer; 2017:757-765.
3. Lerner S, Sternberg C et al. Management of metastatic and invasive bladder cancer. In: Wein A, Kavoussi L, et al., eds. *Campbell-Walsh Urology.* Philadelphia, PA: Elsevier; 2000:2355-2374.
4. Feifer AH, Taylor JM, Tarin TV, et al. Maximizing cure for muscle-invasive bladder cancer: integration of surgery and chemotherapy. *Eur Urol.* 2011;59(6):978-984.
5. Sylvester RJ, van der Meijden AP, Oosterlinck W, et al. Predicting recurrence and progression in individual patients with stage Ta T1 bladder cancer using EORTC risk tables: a combined analysis of 2596 patients from seven EORTC trials. *Eur Urol.* 2006;49(3):466-465.
6. Monn MF, Kaimakliotis H, Pedrosa J, et al. Contemporary bladder cancer: variant histology may be a significant driver of disease. *Urol Oncol.* 2015;33:18.e15-18.e20.
7. Chang, SS, Boorjian SA, et al. Diagnosis and treatment of non-muscle invasive bladder cancer: AUA/SUO Guideline 2016. https://www.auanet.org/education/guidelines/non-muscle-invasive-bladder-cancer.cfm. Accessed April 5, 2017.
8. Meeks JJ, Bellmunt J, Bochner BH, et al. A systematic review of neoadjuvant and adjuvant chemotherapy for muscle-invasive bladder cancer. *Eur Urol.* 2012;62(3):523-533.
9. Zargar H, Espiritu PN, Fairey AS, et al. Multicenter assessment of neoadjuvant chemotherapy for muscle-invasive bladder cancer. *Eur Urol.* 2015;67(2):241-249.
10. Sfakianos JP, Galsky MD. Neoadjuvant chemotherapy in the management of muscle-invasive bladder cancer: bridging the gap between evidence and practice. *Urol Clin N Am.* 2015;42(2):181-187.
11. Grossman HB, Natale RB, Tangen CM, et al. Neoadjuvant chemotherapy plus cystectomy compared with cystectomy alone for locally advanced bladder cancer. *New Engl J Med.* 2003;349(9):859-866.
12. International Collaboration of Trialists. International phase III trial assessing neoadjuvant cisplatin, methotrexate, and vinblastine chemotherapy for muscle-invasive bladder cancer: long-term results of the BA06 30894 Trial. *J Clin Oncol.* 2011;29(16):2171-2177.
13. Malmström PU, Rintala E, Wahlqvist R, et al. Five-year followup of a prospective trial of radical cystectomy and neoadjuvant chemotherapy: Nordic Cystectomy Trial I. The Nordic Cooperative Bladder Cancer Study Group. *J Urol.* 1996;155(6):1903-1906.

14. Advanced Bladder Cancer (ABC) Meta-analysis Collaboration. Neoadjuvant chemotherapy in invasive bladder cancer: update of a systematic review and meta-analysis of individual patient data advanced bladder cancer (ABC) meta-analysis collaboration. *Eur Urol.* August 2005;48(2):202-205.
15. Lavery HJ, Stensland KD, Niegisch G, et al. Pathological T0 following radical cystectomy with or without neoadjuvant chemotherapy: a useful surrogate. *J Urol.* 2014;191(4):898-906.
16. Sonpavde G, Goldman BH, Speights VO, et al. Quality of pathologic response and surgery correlate with survival for patients with completely resected bladder cancer after neoadjuvant chemotherapy. *Cancer.* 2009;115:4104-4109.
17. Shabsigh A, Korets R, Vora KC, et al. Defining early morbidity of radical cystectomy for patients with bladder cancer using a standardized reporting methodology. *Eur Urol.* 2009;55(1):164-174.
18. Liberman D, Lughezzani G, Sun M, et al. Perioperative mortality is significantly greater in septuagenarian and octogenarian patients treated with radical cystectomy for urothelial carcinoma of the bladder. *Urol.* 2011;77:660-668.
19. Neuzillet Y, Soulie M, Larre S, et al. Positive surgical margins and their locations in specimens are adverse prognosis features after radical cystectomy in non-metastatic carcinoma invading bladder muscle: results from a nationwide case–control study. *BJU Int.* 2013:111:1253-1260.
20. Osman Y, Mansour A, El-Tabey N, et al. Value of routine frozen section analysis of urethral margin in male patients undergoing radical cystectomy in predicting prostatic involvement. *Int Urol Nephrol.* 2012;44(6):1721-1725.
21. Stein R, Hohenfellner M, Pahernik S, et al. Urinary diversion–approaches and consequences. *Dtsch Arztebl Int.* 2012;109(38): 617-622.
22. Leow JJ, Martin-Doyle W, Rajagopal PS, et al. Adjuvant chemotherapy for invasive bladder cancer: a 2013 updated systematic review and meta-analysis of randomized trials. *Eur Urol.* 2014;66(1):42-54.
23. Sternberg C, Stoneczna I, Kerst JM, et al. Immediate versus deferred chemotherapy after radical cystectomy in patients with pT3–pT4 or N+ M0 urothelial carcinoma of the bladder (EORTC 30994): an intergroup, open-label, randomised phase 3 trial. *Lancet Oncol.* 2015;16(1):76-86.
24. Herr HW. Transurethral resection of muscle-invasive bladder cancer: 10-year outcome. *J Clin Oncol.* 2001;19(1):89-93.
25. Holzbeierlein JM, Lopez-Corona E, et al. Partial cystectomy: a contemporary review of the Memorial Sloan-Kettering Cancer Center experience and recommendations for patient selection. *J Urol.* 2004;172(3):878-881.

26. van der Steen-Banasik E, Ploeg M, Witjes JA, et al. Brachytherapy versus cystectomy in solitary bladder cancer: a case control, multicentre, East-Netherlands study. *Radiother Oncol.* 2009;93(2):352-357.
27. James ND, Hussain SA, Hall E, et al. Radiotherapy with or without chemotherapy in muscle-invasive bladder cancer. *N Engl J Med.* 2012;366(16):1477-1488.
28. Mak RH, Hunt D, Shipley WU, et al. Long-term outcomes in patients with muscle-invasive bladder cancer after selective bladder-preserving combined-modality therapy: a pooled analysis of Radiation Therapy Oncology Group protocols 8802, 8903, 9506, 9706, 9906, and 0233. *J Clin Oncol.* 2014;32(34):3801-3809.
29. Giacalone N, Clayman R, Shipley W, et al. Long-term outcomes after bladder-preserving combined-modality therapy for patients with muscle-invasive bladder cancer [abstract]. *J Clin Oncol.* 2016;34(suppl 2S). Abstract 398.
30. Mak K, Smith A, Eidelman R, et al. Quality of life in long-term survivors of muscle-invasive bladder cancer. *Int J Radiat Oncol Biol Phys.* 2016;96(5):1028-1036.
31. National Comprehensive Cancer Network. NCCN Guidelines version 2.2016, Bladder Cancer. https://www.nccn.org/professionals/physician_gls/pdf/bladder.pdf. Accessed October 26, 2016.

Treatment of Metastatic Bladder Cancer: Chemotherapy and Checkpoint Inhibitors   26

Jose Pacheco and Teresa Gray Hayes

Please note that due to content overlap, first-line systemic treatment of metastatic bladder cancer was discussed in Chapter 22 on treatment of metastatic urothelial cancer of the upper urinary tract.

SECOND-LINE CHEMOTHERAPY OPTIONS

Second-line chemotherapy options include single agents such as docetaxel, gemcitabine, nab-paclitaxel, pemetrexed, and paclitaxel. Phase 2 trials of these agents demonstrate encouraging overall survival (OS). However, only vinflunine has shown improvement in the second-line setting in a phase 3 trial (1,2) (Table 26.1).

In the few patients who still maintain good organ function and adequate performance status, combination regimens may be considered. One of these combinations is gemcitabine plus paclitaxel. In phase 2 and 3 trials, the overall response rate (ORR) rate ranged from 30% to 70%. The progression free survival (PFS) and OS range from 3.1 to 6.1 months and 8 to 14.4 months, respectively. It is important to realize that in all of these trials it was not clear how many patients had progressed after perioperative therapy for locally advanced disease or first-line therapy in the metastatic setting (1).

Another combination that may be considered is carboplatin plus paclitaxel. In phase 2 trials, the ORR is 16% to 38%. The PFS and OS range from 3.7 to 7.9 months and 6 to 17.3 months, respectively. If patients have demonstrated platinum sensitivity, which some define as relapse more than 6 months from last treatment, then cisplatin-based combination chemotherapy

Table 26.1 Studies of Second-Line, Single-Agent Chemotherapy Options in Advanced and/or Metastatic Urothelial Cancer

Drug	Trial type	Patients (n)	ORR	Median PFS (mo)	Median OS (mo)	Important high-grade AEs
Docetaxel	Phase 2	30	13.3%	N/A	9	Alopecia, anemia, leukopenia, neutropenia, febrile neutropenia/infection, diarrhea, and mucositis
	Phase 2 (RCT)	70	11%	1.6	7.0	
	Phase 2	31	6%	1.4	9.6	
Gemcitabine	Phase 2	35	23%	3.8	5.0	Anemia, leukopenia, neutropenia, and thrombocytopenia
	Phase 2	24	29%	N/A	13	
	Phase 2	30	11%	4.9 (TTP)	8.7 (DSS)	
	Phase 2	46	25%	3.1	12.6	
Nab-Paclitaxel	Phase 2	48	28%	6	10.8	Alopecia and neuropathy
Paclitaxel	Phase 2	14	7%	N/A	N/A	Alopecia, anemia, neutropenia, neutropenic infection, mucositis, and peripheral neuropathy
	Phase 2	31	10%	2.2 (TTP)	7.2	
	Phase 2	45	9%	3 (TTP)	7	
Pemetrexed	Phase 2	47	28%	2.9 (TTP)	9.6	Neutropenia, febrile neutropenia, and thrombocytopenia
	Phase 2	13	8%	N/A	N/A	
Vinflunine	Phase 3 (RCT)	Vinflunine, n = 253 BSC, n = 117	9% 0%	3.0 1.5	6.9, HR 0.77, $P = .036$ 4.3	Anemia, constipation, neutropenia, febrile neutropenia, and thrombocytopenia

AEs, adverse events; BSC, best supportive care; DSS, disease-specific survival; HR, hazard ratio; N/A, not available; ORR, overall response rate; OS, overall survival; PFS, progression free survival; RCT, randomized controlled trial; TTP, time to progression.

high grade: grade ≥ 3 AEs.

Source: Refs. (1,2).

can be considered in the second-line setting. After failure of gemcitabine plus cisplatin (GC) in such patients, standard-dose methotrexate + vinblastine + doxorubicin + cisplatin (sMVAC) has shown ORR of 30%, median PFS of 5.3 months, and median OS of 10.9 months. In a similar population, dose-dense MVAC has shown time to progression (TTP) of 9.6 months and OS of 16.5 months. It is important to note that some patients in these second-line combination studies had locally advanced, unresectable disease (1).

Cisplatin plus paclitaxel has also been evaluated after progression on GC. Of the patients in this phase 2 study, 39% did not have a response to first-line therapy. In this cohort, the ORR was 36%, median TTP was 6.2 months, and median OS was 10.3 months (3). In the National Comprehensive Cancer Network (NCCN) Clinical Practice Guidelines in Oncology (NCCN Guidelines®), there is no standard second-line regimen after progression on first-line cisplatin-based combination chemotherapy. Any of the previously mentioned treatments could be considered, as could other combination regimens or participation in a clinical trial (4).

CHECKPOINT INHIBITORS IN METASTATIC UROTHELIAL CANCER

Immune checkpoint inhibitors (ICIs) include drugs that inhibit the programmed death-1 (PD-1) receptor or programmed death ligand-1 (PD-L1). Multiple ICIs have been evaluated in clinical trials of patients with metastatic urothelial cancer (UC) (5–9) (Table 26.2). There are now two ICIs approved for use in the second-line setting after progression on platinum-based chemotherapy. These approved ICIs are atezolizumab (a PD-L1 inhibitor) and nivolumab (a PD-1 inhibitor) (4). Approval of other ICIs are likely to come soon.

Pembrolizumab is the only ICI at the time of this publication for which a phase 3 trial comparing it to second line chemotherapy (docetaxel, paclitaxel, or vinflunine) has been completed. Pembrolizumab showed significantly improved ORR (21.1% vs 11.4%) and OS (median 10.3 months vs 7.4 months, hazard ratio [HR] 0.73, $P = 0.0002$) when compared to chemotherapy. While there were no significant differences in median PFS,

Table 26.2 Trials of Immune Checkpoint Inhibitors in Advanced Urothelial Cancer

Drug	Target	Trial type	Patients (n)	ORR	PFS	OS	High-grade AEs
Atezolizumab (PD-L1 staining was on immune cells)	PD-L1	II	310	15% (26% for PD-L1 ≥ 5%)	Median 2.1 months (no difference by PD-L1 staining)	Median 7.9 months (11.4 months for PD-L1 ≥ 5%, 1 year OS 48% for this group) 1 year 50.9%	16%
Avelumab (PD-L1+ ≥ 5% on tumor cells)	PD-L1	Ib	44	18.2% (50% for PD-L1+ and 4.3% for PD-L1−)	24 week: 58.3% in PD-L1+, 16.6% PD-L1−		11.3%
Durvalumab (PD-L1+ ≥ 25% on tumor cells or immune cells)	PD-L1	I/II	103	20.4% (29.5% in PD-L1+ and 7.7% in PD-L1−)	N/A	6 months OS 60.3% (PD-L1+ 68.4% and PD-L1− 44.7%)	5.2%
Nivolumab (PD-L1+ was ≥ 1% on tumor cells)	PD-1	I/II	78	24.4% (26% PD-L1 < 1% and 24% PD-L1 ≥ 1%)	2.8 months (PD-L1+ 5.5 months, PD-L1− 2.8 months), 1 year PFS 21%	Median 9.7 months (PD-L1+ 16.2 months, PD-L1− 9.9 months), 1 year OS 46%	22%
Pembrolizumab	PD-1	III RCT	Pembrolizumab, n = 270	21.1%, $P = 0.001$	Median 2.1 months, 1 year 16.8%, HR 0.98, $P = 0.42$	Median 10.3 months, 1 year 43.9%, HR 0.73, $P = 0.002$	15%
Standard of care chemotherapy (docetaxel, paclitaxel or vinflunine)			Chemotherapy, n = 272	11.4%	Median 3.3 months, 1 year 6.2%	Median 7.4 months, 1 year 30.7%	49.4%

AEs, adverse events; N/A, not available; ORR, overall response rate; OS, overall survival; PD-1, programmed death-1; PD-L1, programmed death ligand-1; PFS, progression free survival; RCT, randomized controlled trial.

High grade: grade ≥ 3 AEs.

1 year PFS was longer with pembrolizumab at 16.8% vs 6.2% with chemotherapy (6) (Table 26.2). Phase 3 clinical trials are currently examining other ICIs in comparison to second line chemotherapy in metastatic UC and we are eagerly awaiting their results.

> **KEY POINTS**
>
> - Second-line chemotherapy options include single agents (e.g., docetaxel, gemcitabine, nab-paclitaxel, paclitaxel, pemetrexed, and vinflunine). Select patients may receive combination regimens.
> - In the NCCN Guidelines there is no standard second-line regimen after progression on first-line cisplatin-based combination chemotherapy.
> - Atezolizumab and nivolumab have been approved for use in pretreated patients with advanced, unresectable, or metastatic urothelial cancer. Approval for other ICIs is likely to follow.

REFERENCES

1. Oing C, Rink M, Oechsle K, et al. Second line chemotherapy for advanced and metastatic urothelial carcinoma: vinflunine and beyond—a comprehensive review of the current literature. *J Urol.* 2016;195(2):254-263.
2. Bellmunt J, Théodore C, Demkov T, et al. Phase III trial of vinflunine plus best supportive care compared with best supportive care alone after a platinum-containing regimen in patients with advanced transitional cell carcinoma of the urothelial tract. *J Clin Oncol.* 2003;27(27):4454-4461.
3. Uhm JE, Lim HY, Kim WS, et al. Paclitaxel with cisplatin as salvage treatment for patients with previously treated advanced transitional cell carcinoma of the urothelial tract. *Neoplasia.* 2007;9:18-22.
4. NCCN Clinical Practice Guidelines in Oncology. Bladder Cancer Guidelines Version 2.2017. Referenced with permission from the NCCN Clinical Practice Guidelines in Oncology (NCCN Guidelines®) for Bladder Cancer V.2.2017. © National Comprehensive Cancer Network, Inc. 2017. Available at: www.NCCN.org. Accessed March 22, 2017.
5. Apolo AB, Infante JR, Hamid O, et al. Avelumab (MSB0010718C; anti-PD-L1) in patients with metastatic urothelial carcinoma from

the JAVELIN solid tumor phase Ib trial: analysis of safety, clinical activity, and PD-L1 expression. *J Clin Oncol.* 2016; 34 (Suppl). Abstract 4514.
6. Bellmunt J, de Wit R, Vaughn DJ, et al. Pembrolizumab as Second-Line Therapy for Advanced Urothelial Carcinoma. *N Engl J Med.* March 16, 2017 ;376(11):1015-1026.
7. Powles T, O'Donnell PH, Massard C, et al. Updated efficacy and tolerability of durvalumab in locally advanced or metastatic urothelial carcinoma. *J Clin Oncol.* 2017;35(Suppl 6S) Abstract 286.
8. Rosenberg JE, Hoffman-Centis J, Powles T, et al. Atezolizumab in patients with locally advanced and metastatic urothelial carcinoma who have progressed following treatment with platinum-based chemotherapy: a single-arm, multicenter, phase 2 trial. *Lancet*, 2016;387(10031):1909-1920.
9. Sharma P, Callahan MK, Bono P, et al. Nivolumab monotherapy in recurrent metastatic urothelial carcinoma (CheckMate 032): a multicentre, open-label, two-stage, multi-arm, phase I/II trial. *Lancet Oncol.* 2016;17(11):1590-1598.

Controversies in the Management of Bladder Cancer 27

Jose Pacheco and Teresa Gray Hayes

There are a multitude of issues in the treatment of bladder cancer (BC) without a true management consensus. To aid the reader we have provided some cases that illustrate common and important management questions that are likely to appear in practice.

Case 1: A 53-year-old male presents with T2N0M0 bladder cancer.

Question 1: Do all cases of muscle invasive bladder cancer need radical cystectomy?

National Comprehensive Cancer Network (NCCN) Clinical Practice Guidelines in Oncology (NCCN Guidelines®) state that organ preservation can be considered for patients with T2a to T3 BC. There is no consensus on how to accomplish this. Modalities may include transurethral resection of bladder tumor (TURBT), chemotherapy, radiation and/or partial cystectomy. Bladder preservation is more accepted for nonsurgical candidates, although it still may be underutilized (1). However, for those patients who do not desire radical cystectomy (RC) and are otherwise surgical candidates, the physician recommendations are challenging. Part of this dilemma is that there is a high rate of discordance between clinical tumor stage and pathological stage at the time of RC. Because of this controversy, the NCCN recommends that for surgical candidates, bladder preservation options should only be chosen in the context of clinical trials or if patients refuse surgery (1).

Of the preservation options mentioned, chemoradiation has the most supportive data. TURBT alone should only be considered in select cases with tumors less than 2 cm, minimal muscle invasion, no in situ disease, no palpable mass, and no hydronephrosis. Chemotherapy alone is considered inadequate, as the pathologic complete response (CR) rate in the bladder is low. Similarly, radiation alone is not recommended unless patients cannot tolerate chemotherapy, as results are inferior to those of combined modality treatment. Chemoradiation should only be considered in potential surgical candidates if complete resection can be obtained with TURBT. The category 2A recommendations for chemotherapy given as part of combined modality treatment in this situation are: cisplatin, cisplatin + 5-fluorouracil (5-FU), cisplatin + paclitaxel, and 5-FU + Mitomycin C (1).

Six Radiation Therapy Oncology Group (RTOG) studies have examined chemoradiation in bladder preservation. Five of them were phase 2 trials and one was a phase 3 trial. In a meta-analysis of these trials, the 5-year- and 10-year overall survival (OS) were 57% and 36%, respectively. Disease-specific survival, muscle-invasive local-regional failure, nonmuscle invasive local regional failure, and distant metastasis at 5 and 10 years were 71% and 65%, 13% and 14%, 31% and 36%, and 31% and 35%, respectively. Some of these trials utilized a neoadjuvant (NA) chemotherapy approach prior to concurrent chemoradiation; however, this has not been shown to provide additional benefit. In these trials, there were no excess high-grade acute or long-term toxicities (2).

A meta-analysis of retrospective and prospective studies examining chemoradiation and bladder preservation in muscle invasive BC was recently published. There were 13,396 patients. It is suggested that this approach may actually have a survival advantage compared to RC upfront or after NA chemotherapy. The 5-year OS rate for the bladder preservation group was 57%, compared to 52% (51% for RC alone and 53% for RC + chemotherapy) in those who did not undergo bladder preservation ($P = .04$, hazard ratio [HR] 1.22 for RC) (3).

It is important to remember that these bladder preservation strategies are for the most part dependent on having a clinical CR to combined modality therapy. Since the survival outcomes are in many cases similar or better than those who have undergone RC, what may be happening is that this approach selects for patients with biologically less aggressive tumors that are more responsive to chemoradiation. To further understand the true effect of these bladder-preservation strategies, we need to await the results of further trials where patients who attain a clinical CR to NA combined modality treatment are randomized to either bladder preservation or RC.

Case 2: A 67-year-old male presented with 3 months of gross hematuria. He was found to have T4bN1M0 urothelial carcinoma of the bladder. He was deemed not a surgical candidate because of nodal involvement and T4b disease.

Question 2: After NA therapy, could he become an operative candidate?

Bladder cancer that is clinically T4b and/or has positive lymph nodes is generally considered unresectable, and the median OS without surgery is a little over a year. However, the NCCN Guidelines® suggest that in select cases RC may be considered in these patients after NA therapy. In these cases, the guidelines suggest chemotherapy and/or radiation may be used in the NA setting (1).

Small cohort and retrospective studies have suggested that in certain patients with T4 disease and/or clinically positive lymph nodes undergoing RC after NA chemotherapy, improved survival may be achieved. One such retrospective study looked at the response to NA chemotherapy in 304 patients who were initially felt to be unresectable due to clinically positive lymph nodes and who received mainly cisplatin-based regimens followed by RC. Interestingly, the median OS for the whole cohort was 22 months, although the median follow-up was only 13 months. Forty-eight percent of patients achieved pN0 disease. For those with pN0 disease, the median OS was 71 to 84 months, depending on the initial number of clinically positive nodes (4). When interpreting this and other retrospective analyses, it is important to keep in mind that these were nonrandomized, very select patient populations. Such studies may not be representative of all patients with clinically positive lymph nodes and the particular study discussed in detail earlier did not include patients with T4b disease.

Case 3: After NA chemotherapy, a patient is to undergo RC. His initial stage was T3N0M0.

Question 3: What extent of lymphadenectomy should the patient receive at the time of surgery?
According to the NCCN Guidelines, pelvic lymphadenectomy is an essential component in the surgical treatment of bladder cancer. An extended pelvic lymphadenectomy that includes the common iliac and sometimes the lower para-aortic nodes is associated with improved survival (1). However, there is some controversy as to how extensive such lymphadenectomy really needs to be, since the supporting evidence is retrospective or nonrandomized prospective data. Our patient should, at a minimum, undergo a bilateral pelvic lymph node dissection that includes the obturator fossa, internal and external iliac basin, the fossa of Marcille, and the lymph nodes around the common iliac artery. However, the optimal superior extent of such dissection (ureteropelvic junction or aortic bifurcation) is not known. Additionally, there is no specific number of lymph nodes that should be removed (5).

Case 4: A 64-year-old female is diagnosed with a high grade T1N0M0 transitional cell carcinoma of the urothelium. She undergoes a repeat TURBT 6 weeks after the initial one and is found to have residual nonmuscle invasive disease.

Question 4: Should this patient now receive treatment with intravesicular Bacillus Calmette-Guérin (BCG) or RC?
The NCCN Guidelines state that for residual disease in this setting, intravesicular BCG is a category 1 option. A second option, which carries a 2A recommendation, is to perform RC (1). Performing an RC in these patients instead of intravesicular therapy is controversial because of the morbidity associated with the procedure. Part of the impetus for this approach is that there is a significant amount of clinical understaging in BC. This understaging may be part of why some reports suggest that as many as 53% of high-grade T1 lesions will progress to muscle invasive disease. Additionally, some data suggest that intravesicular BCG may not delay progression in these patients, as an estimated 34% will die of BC within 15 years (6). However, there has been no trial showing a survival benefit to RC over intravesicular therapy in these patients.

> **KEY POINTS**
>
> - Bladder preservation can be considered in select patients with T2a to T3 bladder cancer, but should only be done if patients refuse surgery, are not surgical candidates, or as part of a clinical trial.
> - One can consider RC in select cases of nonmetastatic T4b or node-positive bladder cancer after NA therapy.

REFERENCES

1. Bladder Cancer Guidelines Version 2.2017. Referenced with permission from the NCCN Clinical Practice Guidelines in Oncology (NCCN Guidelines®) for Bladder Cancer V.2.2017. ©National Comprehensive Cancer Network, Inc., 2017, all rights reserved. Accessed March 22, 2017. To view the most recent and complete version of the guideline, go online to NCCN.org. NATIONAL COMPREHENSIVE CANCER NETWORK®, NCCN®, NCCN GUIDELINES®, and all other NCCN Content are trademarks owned by the National Comprehensive Cancer Network, Inc.
2. Mak RH, Hunt D, Shipley WU, et al. Long-term outcomes in patients with muscle-invasive bladder cancer after selective bladder-preserving combined-modality therapy: a pooled analysis of Radiation Therapy Oncology Group protocols 8802, 8903, 9506, 9706, 9906, and 0233. *J Clin Oncol.* 2014;32(34):3801-3909.
3. Arcangeli G, Strigari L, Arcangeli S. Radical cystectomy versus organ-sparing versus organ-sparing trimodality treatment in muscle-invasive bladder cancer: a systematic review of clinical trials. *Crit Rev Oncol Hematol.* 2015;95(3):387-396.
4. Zargar-Shoshtari K, Zargar H, Lotan Y, et al. A multi-institutional analysis of outcomes of patients with clinically node positive urothelial bladder cancer treated with induction chemotherapy and radical cystectomy. *J Urol.* 2016;195(1):53-59.
5. Tilki D, Brausi M, Colombo R, et al. Lymphadenectomy for bladder cancer at the time of radical cystectomy. *Eur Urol.* 2013;64(2):266-276.
6. Cookson MS, Herr HW, Zhang ZF, et al. The treated natural history of high-risk superficial bladder cancer: 15-year outcome. *J Urol.* 1997;158(1):62-67.

Bladder Cancer Surveillance and Survivorship 28

Bethany R. Desroches and Jennifer Marie Taylor

SURVIVAL

As described in the preceding sections, bladder cancer is the fourth most common cancer in U.S. men, although not even the 10th most common cancer in U.S. women (1). For all stages combined, the 5-year relative survival is 77%. Survival decreases to 70% at 10 years, and 65% at 14 years after diagnosis, contrasting with only 10% to 15% of patients alive 5 years after the diagnosis of metastatic disease. With an estimated 74,000 new cases diagnosed in 2016, there will be 17,900 deaths, consistent with the excellent survival of low-stage disease.

There are estimated to be over 500,000 patients alive in the United States living with bladder cancer. With a median age at diagnosis of 65 years, medical comorbidities are more common than in a younger population. These factors, as well as disease-specific elements of stage, grade, and histology, all impact the discussion of future surveillance and care. Advanced age predicts greater risk of other-cause mortality; locally advanced or distant disease most strongly predicts worse cancer-specific survival. Involvement of a multidisciplinary team can benefit a patient's long-term survival. By integrating care, providers can encourage the patient to pursue a healthy lifestyle, decrease weight if indicated, and to avoid or quit any tobacco use or exposure.

NONMUSCLE INVASIVE BLADDER CANCER

Recurrence: The approximate probability of recurrence in 5 years varies from 50% for low-grade Ta to 60% to 90% for Tis, with risk of progression ranging from 5% in low-risk Ta disease and approaching 50% for high-risk disease. The most important prognostic factors for disease progression and disease-specific survival are stage and grade. For patients with high-grade nonmuscle invasive bladder cancer (NMIBC), the cancer-specific survival has been shown to be 70% to 85% at 10 years (2). While there is a high risk of recurrence (up to 55%) for low-grade Ta lesions, only 6% of these progress to high-grade or invasive disease (3). In contrast, high-grade T1 lesions will recur at an elevated rate (45%), with 1- and 5-year disease-progression rates of 11.4% and 19.8%, respectively.

All patients with diagnosed NMIBC must understand that surveillance is the key to proactive monitoring and identification of recurrence. The American Urological Association (AUA) NMIBC guidelines provide a framework for risk groups that informs treatment recommendations, recurrence risk, and surveillance (see Chapter 24).

Surveillance: Guidelines are available from National Comprehensive Cancer Network (NCCN) and the AUA. First cystoscopy after resection is recommended at 3 months, with cytology, and then every 3 to 6 months and at increasing intervals thereafter, depending on risk stratification. Further, upper tract imaging is recommended at 1- to 2-year intervals for intermediate- and high-risk patients. Imaging should be contrast enhanced with delayed phase images, such as CT or magnetic resonance (MR) urogram. Patients with allergy or renal insufficiency may undergo noncontrast CT or ultrasound with retrograde pyelograms. Bone scan, PET/CT, and brain imaging are not recommended for routine monitoring.

MUSCLE INVASIVE BLADDER CANCER

Recurrence: Risks of disease recurrence and progression depend on treatment given and pathologic details. High-risk features which can be identified at resection or cystectomy include lymphovascular invasion, extravesical extension of disease, node positivity, presence of carcinoma in situ (CIS), aberrant histology, and positive soft tissue margins at cystectomy. Following cystectomy, the site of relapse will be local in 10% to 30% of cases and distant in 70% to 90%. The European Organization for Research and Treatment of Cancer (EORTC) estimates that patients with muscle invasive bladder cancer (MIBC) have 5-year survival rates of between 30% and 60%.

Surveillance: The NCCN guidelines recommend chest imaging in early stages of disease and disease follow-up with chest x-ray or CT if there are or were previously observed questionable changes in the thorax. PET/CT may be performed if not previously done to rule out metastases in selected patients. Upper tract imaging should be offered at 3 to 6 month intervals for 2 years, and then at 1-year intervals. In cases of definitive whole bladder radiation or the rare case of partial cystectomy, bladder surveillance with cystoscopy is necessary. The presence of residual or recurrent-invasive disease should prompt a discussion of salvage cystectomy if appropriate. With known advanced or metastatic disease, serial axial imaging of chest, abdomen, and pelvis can be done by PET/CT, standard CT, or MRI.

After radical cystectomy, surveillance must include imaging, lab studies, and urine cytology to monitor the upper urothelial tracts and urethra. Results of a meta-analysis of 13,185 patients who underwent cystectomy had a recurrence of upper tract pathology of between 0.75% and 6.4% (4). However, it is important to note that urine cytology only discovered 7% of these recurrences and upper urinary tract imaging detected 30%, so the physician must use clinical judgment to pursue further treatment if hematuria or other clinical signs point toward the need for further investigation. Urethral wash cytology should also be performed, particularly in those with high-risk features such as prostatic urethral disease or concomitant CIS. Monitoring of renal function with creatinine is important, as changes could indicate an anatomic issue such as a ureteral stricture. Further, if ileum was used for the bladder reconstruction, serum B12 levels should be screened annually. The key side effects of systemic treatments such as chemotherapy must also be monitored during and after therapy.

SURVIVORSHIP

Quality of life is a key outcome for patients receiving these treatments. Some patients face anxiety, fear, and depression, and these diagnoses may impact their ability to return for follow-up appointments and tests. There is clear benefit to working with a multidisciplinary team, including psychologists and social workers, to ensure that each bladder cancer survivor will be adherent with first their treatment and later their surveillance and follow-up visits.

Diagnostic and therapeutic interventions can affect urinary and sexual function, as well as body image. These factors should be discussed before surgery and followed prospectively at subsequent visits in patients who have undergone resection, intravesical therapy, radiation, or cystectomy. As patients are at times reluctant to bring up these issues, the provider should question the patient directly for impairment or distress. Validated questionnaires such as the International Prostate Symptom Score (IPSS) and bladder cancer specific tools, such as the EORTC-Quality of Life Questionnaire (QLQ), can assist in these discussions.

Overall, for survivors with no known disease, providers must monitor for recurrence and for sequelae of treatments (both medical and surgical). Multiple organizations provide guidelines for long-term evaluation of patients after treatment of their bladder cancer (see general references listed). The 5-year relative survival rate for bladder cancers diagnosed during 2005 to 2011 was 69%, up from 49% during the period 1975 to 1977 (1). Many specialists are excited about the potential gains to be made with new immunotherapy choices, and 2016 marked the first time in over 20 years a new drug was approved by the Food and Drug Administration (FDA) for bladder cancer.

The goals remain to treat the initial cancer appropriately with selected surgical and medical therapy; screen for recurrence; provide psychosocial and quality of life support; and work in multidisciplinary teams to optimize care for these patients.

KEY POINTS

- Coordination of posttreatment care is important between primary physicians and specialists.
- Expectations and survivorship issues vary by type of disease and treatment.
- Screening for recurrence and secondary cancers should continue lifelong.

REFERENCES

1. American Cancer Society. Cancer Facts & Figures 2016. http://www.cancer.org/acs/groups/content/@research/documents/document/acspc-047079.pdf. Accessed December 22, 2016.
2. Leblanc B, Duclos AJ, Benard F, et al. Long-term followup of initial Ta grade 1 transitional cell carcinoma of the bladder. *J Urol.* 1999;162(6):1946-1950.
3. American Urological Association. Diagnosis and treatment of non-muscle invasive bladder cancer: AUA/SUO Guideline–AUA/SUO 2016. https://www.auanet.org/education/guidelines/non-muscle-invasive-bladder-cancer.cfm. Accessed December 22, 2016.
4. Picozzi S, Ricci C, Gaeta M, et al. Upper urinary tract recurrence following radical cystectomy for bladder cancer: a meta-analysis on 13,185 patients. *J Urol.* 2012;188:2046-2054.

RECOMMENDED READING

- Cancer Facts & Figures 2016, American Cancer Society
- Diagnosis and Treatment of Non-Muscle Invasive Bladder Cancer: AUA/SUO Guideline–AUA/SUO 2016
- European Journal Of Urology Guidelines: Bladder Cancer: Muscle Invasive and Metastatic
- European Journal Of Urology Guidelines: Non-Invasive Bladder Cancer
- National Comprehensive Cancer Network (NCCN) Guidelines Version 1.2017–Bladder Cancer 12/21/16

TESTICULAR CANCER

Seminomas 29

Mehmet Akce and Teresa Gray Hayes

INTRODUCTION

Testicular cancer is 1%–2% of all tumors in men between the ages of 15 and 35 (1). In 2015, there were an estimated 8,430 new testicular cancer cases in the United States, accounting for 380 deaths from testicular cancer (2). Testicular cancer classically presents with a painless testicular mass, which should be evaluated urgently. The standard work up of testicular cancer includes a routine complete blood count with differential, complete metabolic panel, and testicular ultrasound. The first step of treatment in testicular cancer is orchiectomy. Inguinal orchiectomy is the standard of care, and transscrotal orchiectomy should never be performed when malignancy is suspected. Beta-human chorionic gonadotropin (B-HCG), alpha-fetoprotein (AFP), and lactate dehydrogenase (LDH) are the serum tumor markers (STMs) in testicular cancer, useful in diagnosis, prognosis, and staging. However, none of the STMs are specific for testicular cancer. STMs should be checked prior to orchiectomy and repeated following orchiectomy.

HISTOLOGY

Germ cell tumors (GCTs) comprise 95% of all primary testicular cancers. GCTs are divided into seminomas and nonseminomas. Sixty percent of all GCTs of the testis are seminomas (1). A diagnosis of pure seminoma requires both histologic evidence of seminoma and a normal AFP level, as pure seminomas do not produce AFP. Patients with elevated AFP despite apparently pure seminoma histology should be evaluated carefully for the presence of a nonseminomatous component of the tumor. They should be treated as nonseminomas unless a nontumor related cause is found for the increased AFP.

SERUM TUMOR MARKERS

STMs are an essential part of the tumor, node, metastasis (TNM) staging of testicular cancer. The half-lives of AFP and beta HCG are 7 and 3 days, respectively. Proper staging of testicular cancer is done after radical orchiectomy. STMs are expected to decline according to their half-lives once the tumor has been surgically removed.

STAGING

There are three stages of testicular cancer. In stage I testicular cancer, the tumor is confined to the testis or spermatic cord with normal STMs. In stage II testicular cancer, retroperitoneal (RP) lymph nodes are involved and the size of the RP lymph nodes with normal or mildly elevated STMs define stage II A, B, or C (RP lymph node <2 cm defines stage IIA, 2 to 5 cm defines stage IIB, and >5 cm defines stage IIC). Stage III testicular cancer is characterized by the presence of distant organ metastasis, pelvic lymph node involvement, or RP lymph node involvement with moderately/highly elevated STMs (Table 29.1) (3).

For stage I or II, tumor markers cannot be highly elevated. Very high tumor markers are consistent with stage III seminoma. The persistence of STMs after treatment of stage I seminoma implies the presence of micrometastatic disease and is treated as stage III. Based on STMs and primary and metastatic tumor site, the International Germ Cell Cancer Collaborative Group (IGCCCG) system categorized metastatic GCTs into good risk, intermediate risk, and poor risk groups, with 5-year survival rates of 91%, 79%, and 48%, respectively (4). There is no high risk seminoma, only good risk or intermediate risk seminoma. Metastatic disease to organs other than lungs is considered intermediate risk seminoma, and the rest of seminomas are good risk disease.

Table 29.1 Staging for Testicular Cancer

Stage	Tumor size	Lymph node	Metastasis	Tumor markers
0	Carcinoma in situ	N0: no regional lymph node metastases	M0: no distant metastasis	Marker study levels within normal limits
I	Any pathologic T stage IA (pT1): limited to testis without LVI, may invade tunica albuginea but not tunica vaginalis IB (pT2): limited to testis and epididymis with LVI, or extends through tunica albuginea with involvement of tunica vaginalis or (pT3): invades spermatic cord with or without LVI or (pT4): invades scrotum with or without LVI	N0: no regional lymph node metastases	M0: no distant metastasis	Marker study levels normal, not available or not performed
IS	Any pathologic T stage	No regional lymph node metastases	M0: no distant metastasis	Tumor markers elevated
II	Any pathologic T stage	Regional lymph node metastases IIA (N1): Lymph node mass ≤2 cm, or multiple nodes, none >2 cm; IIB (N2): Lymph node mass >2 cm and ≤5 cm, or multiple nodes, none >5 cm; IIC (N3): Lymph node mass >5 cm	M0: no distant metastasis	S0: tumor markers normal, or S1: LDH <1.5× normal and hCG <5,000 and AFP <1,000

(continued)

Table 29.1 Staging for Testicular Cancer (continued)

Stage	Tumor size	Lymph node	Metastasis	Tumor markers
III	Any pathologic T stage	Any N	M1: distant metastasis	± Tumor markers elevated
IIIA	Any pathologic T stage	Any N	M1A: nonregional nodal or pulmonary metastasis	S0 or S1
IIIB	Any pathologic T stage	Any N	M0 or M1A	S2: LDH 1.5–10 × normal or hCG 5,000–50,000 or AFP 1,000–10,000
IIIC	Any pathologic T stage	Any N	M0, M1A, or M1B (distant metastasis other than to regional nodes or lung)	S3: LDH > 10 × normal or hCG > 50,000 or AFP > 10,000 or any S with M1B

AFP, alpha-fetoprotein; hCG, human chorionic gonadotropin; LDH, lactate dehydrogenase; LVI, lymphovascular invasion.

Source: Adapted from Ref. (3). American Joint Committee on Cancer. Testis. In: Amin MB, Edge SB, Greene FL, et al., eds., AJCC Cancer Staging Manual, 8th Edition. Chicago: Springer, 2017:727–735.

EARLY STAGE SEMINOMA

Stage I Seminoma

Patients present with stage I disease in 80% of cases. There are three standard treatment options in stage I seminoma following radical inguinal orchiectomy: Active surveillance, adjuvant radiotherapy, or adjuvant chemotherapy with one or two cycles of carboplatin. Any of these three strategies results in an almost 100% disease free survival in stage I seminoma (1,5). Active surveillance is the preferred approach per National Comprehensive Cancer Network (NCCN) guidelines, and the pros and cons of each treatment option should be discussed with the patient (6). The reported relapse rates ranged between 1.8 and 8.6 after one or two cycles of carboplatin (7). The updated results of a randomized trial of one cycle of carboplatin versus radiotherapy in 1,477 patients with stage I seminoma reported a 5-year relapse rate of 5.3% for the carboplatin arm and 4% for the radiotherapy arm (8). The relapse rate is between 13% and 19% for active surveillance (1,5). An increased risk of secondary malignancies and cardiovascular diseases should be noted as long-term risks of radiation therapy in the management of early stage seminoma (1). Sperm banking should be discussed with the patients prior to chemotherapy due to an increased risk of infertility.

Surveillance

CT abdomen/pelvis is the recommended imaging modality for surveillance of early stage seminomas. Time intervals depend on whether adjuvant chemotherapy or radiotherapy was given following radical orchiectomy. Chest x-ray is utilized as clinically indicated. STMs have low utility in active surveillance for stage I seminoma, and the American Society of Clinical Oncology recommended against the use of STMs in surveillance of stage I seminoma (9).

Relapse

With active surveillance, more than 90% of relapses occur in the first 3 years. After adjuvant therapy, 99% of relapses occur within the first 3 years. For patients who relapse during surveillance, treatment is still given with curative intent. Para-aortic lymph nodes are the most common sites of relapse. Radiation therapy can cure nonbulky (<5 cm) relapse in more than 90% of patients (1). Three cycles of bleomycin, etoposide, and cisplatin (BEP) or four cycles of etoposide and cisplatin (EP) are typically used for large, bulky relapses (10). Relapses may occur in a supradiaphragmatic site after adjuvant radiotherapy, and cisplatin-based chemotherapy is used in this setting. Relapses occurring in RP lymph nodes after adjuvant chemotherapy can be treated with salvage radiation therapy or cisplatin-based salvage chemotherapy.

Stage II Seminoma

Clinical or pathological abdominal and/or pelvic lymph involvement indicates stage II seminoma. At initial presentation, 15% to 20% of cases are stage II (11). The size of the lymph node involvement determines stages IIA, B, and C. Treatment modalities include adjuvant chemotherapy or radiotherapy. The optimal treatment modality depends on the extent of lymph node involvement. Essentially, stage IIA disease can be treated with radiation therapy or chemotherapy, and stage IIB and stage IIC are treated with chemotherapy only. Radiation therapy to para-aortic and ipsilateral iliac lymph nodes with 30 Gy is the preferred dose for stage IIA seminoma per NCCN guidelines, and 36 Gy can be considered for nonbulky stage IIB disease (6). Single agent carboplatin is not adequate treatment for stage IIA and B disease, as the phase II clinical trial conducted by the German Testicular Cancer Study Group revealed only an 81% (88/108 patients) complete response rate in patients with stage IIA and B seminoma after three or four cycles of carboplatin AUC 7, respectively (12). Cisplatin-based combination chemotherapy is recommended for stage IIA disease, especially in the setting of multiple lymph node involvement, and is the preferred approach for stages IIB and IIC disease. Three cycles of BEP or four cycles of EP are typical chemotherapy combinations. The disease specific survival rate exceeds 95% in stage II seminoma, regardless of the initial treatment modality (11).

Residual Mass

A residual mass following the primary treatment with combination chemotherapy or radiotherapy is one of the challenges in the management of stage II seminoma. The majority of these masses include necrotic or fibrotic tissue, but a few contain tumor. Although the size of the residual mass may be helpful to determine the next step of action, PET scan can be instrumental in guiding clinical decisions. Surveillance or PET scan can be considered if the size of the residual mass is less than 3 cm versus greater than 3 cm, respectively. If the PET scan is negative, surveillance can be considered. If it is positive, retroperitoneal lymph node dissection (RPLND) or second line chemotherapy are options. Surveillance strategy includes periodic history and physical examinations, CT abdomen/pelvis, and chest x-ray. The time intervals of the imaging studies depend on the bulkiness of disease and staging as outlined in NCCN guidelines (6).

LATE STAGE SEMINOMA

Stage III Seminoma

Nonregional lymph node or distant organ metastasis indicates stage III seminoma. As mentioned earlier, metastasis to distant organs other than lungs is considered intermediate risk disease; all other seminomas are considered good risk disease. Chemotherapy is the treatment of choice in late stage seminoma, and the risk group determines the number of chemotherapy cycles. Standard chemotherapy options are three cycles of BEP or four cycles of EP for good risk disease, whereas four cycles of BEP is recommended for intermediate risk disease. VIP (etoposide, ifosfamide, and cisplatin) can be used in patients who cannot receive bleomycin. Seminomas are highly chemosensitive, and cure rates exceed 80% in disseminated good risk seminomas in the first-line chemotherapy setting (13).

Relapse

The majority of relapses occur in the first 2 years of treatment. Late relapse for seminomas is rare. Most trials evaluating salvage chemotherapy regimens in relapsed or disseminated GCT included more nonseminomatous GCTs than pure seminomas. However, chemotherapy regimens are similar for seminomas and nonseminomatous GCTs in the second line setting. Second line chemotherapy options are VeIP (vinblastine, ifosfamide, and cisplatin), TIP (paclitaxel, ifosfamide, and cisplatin), and high dose chemotherapy (HDC) followed by autologous stem cell transplant. Sustained complete response rates are between 24% and 25% for VeIP, 38% to 63% for TIP, and 40% to 50% for HDC (13). Palliative chemotherapy options for refractory patients include gemcitabine, oxaliplatin, paclitaxel, or irinotecan as a single agent or in combination, as well as single agent oral etoposide (6,14).

> **KEY POINTS**
>
> - The diagnosis of pure seminoma requires both histologic evidence of seminoma and a normal AFP level.
> - If testicular malignancy is suspected, inguinal rather than transscrotal orchiectomy should be performed.
> - Staging is determined by tumor size and spread and the level of STMs.
> - Depending on the stage and risk factors, seminomas are treated with orchiectomy alone, adjuvant chemotherapy or radiotherapy, or combination chemotherapy.
> - Seminomas have a high primary cure rate, and relapsed seminomas are still potentially curable.

REFERENCES

1. Chung P, Warde P. Contemporary management of stage I and II seminoma. *Curr Urol Rep.* 2013;14(5):525-533.
2. Siegel RL, Miller KD, Jemal A. Cancer statistics, 2015. *CA: Cancer J Clin.* 2015;65(1):5-29.
3. American Joint Committee on Cancer. Testis. In: Amin MB, Edge SB, Greene FL, et al., eds. AJCC Cancer Staging Manual, 8th Edition. Chicago: Springer, 2017:727-735.
4. Wilkinson PM, Read G. International Germ Cell Consensus Classification: a prognostic factor-based staging system for metastatic germ cell cancers. International Germ Cell Cancer Collaborative Group. *J Clin Oncol.* 1997;15(2):594-603.
5. Pearce SM, Liauw SL, Eggener SE. Management of low-stage testicular seminoma. *Urol Clin N Am.* 2015;42(3):287–298.
6. NCCN. Clinical practice guidelines in oncology: testicular cancer. V1.2017. https://www.nccn.org/professionals/physician_gls/pdf/testicular.pdf. Accessed November 11, 2016.

7. Chung P, Mayhew LA, Warde P, et al. Management of stage I seminomatous testicular cancer: a systematic review. *Clin Oncol.* 2010;22(1):6-16.
8. Oliver, RTD, Mead GM, Rustin GJ, et al. Randomized trial of carboplatin versus radiotherapy for stage I seminoma: mature results on relapse and contralateral testis cancer rates in MRC TE19/EORTC 30982 study (ISRCTN27163214). *J Clin Oncol.* 2011;29(8):957-962.
9. Gilligan TD, Seidenfeld J, Basch E, et al. American Society of Clinical Oncology Clinical Practice Guideline on uses of serum tumor markers in adult males with germ cell tumors. *J Clin Oncol.* 2010;28(20):3388-3404.
10. Ehrlich Y, Margel D, Lubin MA, et al. Advances in the treatment of testicular cancer. *Translational Androl Urol.* 2015;4(3):381–390.
11. Chung, PW, Bedard P. Stage II seminomas and nonseminomas. *Hematol Oncol Clin N Am.* 2011;25(3):529-541.
12. Krege S, Boergermann C, Baschek R, et al. Single agent carboplatin for CS IIA/B testicular seminoma. A phase II study of the German Testicular Cancer Study Group (GTCSG). *Ann Oncol.* 2006;17(2):276-280.
13. Voss MH, Feldman DR, Bosl GJ, et al. A review of second-line chemotherapy and prognostic models for disseminated germ cell tumors. *Hematol Oncol Clinics N Am.* 2011;25(3):557-576.
14. Calabrò F, Albers P, Bokemeyer C, et al. The contemporary role of chemotherapy for advanced testis cancer: a systematic review of the literature. *Eur Urol.* 2012;61(6):1212-1221.

Nonseminomatous Germ Cell Tumors: Early Stage, Late Stage 30

Ryan Yates and Martha Pritchett Mims

NONSEMINOMA

Compared with seminomas, nonseminomas are more likely to present with distant disease, are more radioresistant, and are more likely to be associated with elevated tumor markers, specifically alpha fetoprotein (AFP). Men with pure seminomas never have elevations in AFP, and a histologically defined seminoma in the context of an elevated AFP is considered a mixed germ cell tumor and should be treated as a nonseminoma.

The management of nonseminomatous germ cell tumors (NSGCTs) is dependent upon stage and tumor marker elevation. Stages I and IIA or IIB NSGCTs without significant tumor marker elevation are characterized as early stage disease, whereas late stage, or advanced disease, is defined as stage IIC, stage III, or any stage disease with significant postorchiectomy tumor marker elevation. Staging and risk classification (for advanced disease) is determined based on guidelines from the American Joint Committee on Cancer (AJCC) and International Germ Cell Cancer Consensus Group (IGCCCG) (1,2).

EARLY STAGE DISEASE

Initial management, as in almost all testicular germ cell tumors, includes radical inguinal orchiectomy. Postorchiectomy tumor marker evaluation, chest radiograph, and abdominal and pelvic CT scan are also necessary to exclude more advanced disease.

- **Stage I NSGCT**

  If stage I disease is confirmed, management options following orchiectomy include active surveillance, nerve-sparing retroperitoneal lymph node dissection (RPLND), or adjuvant chemotherapy. Approximately 75% of patients with clinical stage I disease are cured with initial orchiectomy (3). Thus, adjuvant treatment (RPLND or chemotherapy) represents overtreatment in the majority of patients. Unfortunately, it is difficult to determine which patients are at the highest risk of relapse and have the most to gain from adjuvant treatment. Several risk factors for recurrence have emerged including lymphovascular invasion (LVI), predominance of an embryonal carcinoma component in the primary tumor, and pathologic T3 or T4 tumors. Men with LVI-positive tumors have relapse rates of approximately 50%, whereas men with LVI-negative tumors have relapse rates closer to 15% (4). The optimal approach to management is controversial but depends on an assessment of the likelihood of relapse, patient preference, potential for treatment toxicity, and the ability of a patient to adhere to surveillance. For men who are interested in fertility preservation, sperm banking should be performed prior to treatment with RPLND or chemotherapy.

  - **Stage IA NSGCT**

    Recommended management options include active surveillance and nerve-sparing RPLND (5). While the overall survival of patients exceeds 95% for either option, strict adherence to surveillance guidelines is crucial, as numerous studies have shown that 20% to 30% of patients who choose active surveillance experience relapse and ultimately require chemotherapy (3). Access to a urologist with extensive experience performing RPLNDs is crucial for patients who wish to proceed with this option.

    Following nerve-sparing RPLND, the decision to give adjuvant chemotherapy is based on the extent of nodal involvement. Surveillance is preferred for patients with pN0 or pN1 disease (which would correlate with stage IA disease), while chemotherapy is preferred for patients with more extensive nodal involvement (pN2 or pN3). Two cycles of etoposide/cisplatin (EP) or bleomycin/

etoposide/cisplatin (BEP) are sufficient for most patients with pN2 disease, while four cycles of EP or three cycles of BEP are recommended for patients with pN3 disease (5).

- **Stage IB NSGCT**

  Chemotherapy or nerve-sparing RPLND is recommended by the National Comprehensive Cancer Network (NCCN) after initial orchiectomy. Several studies support the efficacy of two cycles of adjuvant BEP, although benefit from one cycle of BEP has also been established for patients unable to tolerate the toxicity of multiple cycles of chemotherapy (6). If nerve-sparing RPLND is performed, determination of the need for adjuvant chemotherapy is based on nodal involvement, similar to patients with stage IA disease.

- **Stage II NSGCT**

  Stage II disease refers to cancers that have spread to the retroperitoneal lymph nodes. Stage II disease can be defined clinically (based on imaging alone) or pathologically (based on lymph node involvement at the time of RPLND). Of note, pelvic or inguinal lymph node involvement is considered distant disease and is indicative of advanced, stage III disease.

  - **Stage IIA NSGCT**

    Treatment depends upon the postorchiectomy tumor markers. Adjuvant chemotherapy (four cycles of EP or three cycles of BEP) or primary nerve-sparing RPLND are both reasonable options for patients with normal postorchiectomy tumor markers. However, chemotherapy is preferred in patients with elevated tumor markers. In patients who undergo primary chemotherapy, subsequent management depends upon repeat CT scan to evaluate lymph node response to treatment. Bilateral nerve-sparing RPLND is often performed for residual lesions greater than 1 cm, whereas surveillance is most often preferred for patients with residual lesions less than 1 cm or normal tumor markers. In patients who undergo primary RPLND, the decision to proceed with adjuvant chemotherapy depends on the extent of nodal involvement. As noted earlier, no chemotherapy is recommended for pN0 or pN1 disease.

- **Stage IIB NSGCT**

  Proper management depends on postorchiectomy tumor markers and radiographic findings. In the absence of tumor marker elevation, CT findings are used to direct treatment. If nodal involvement is confined to the retroperitoneal lymphatic drainage sites, options are to perform nerve-sparing RPLND followed by chemotherapy based on the degree of nodal involvement, as previously described, or to proceed directly with chemotherapy (four cycles of EP or three cycles of BEP) followed by RPLND or surveillance. Primary chemotherapy versus primary RPLND have comparable outcomes (relapse-free survival close to 98%) but with different side effects and toxicity (7). For patients with lymph node metastases outside the primary lymphatic drainage site, chemotherapy (four cycles of EP or three cycles of BEP) is recommended followed by nerve-sparing RPLND or surveillance (5).

- **Stage I and II NSGCT With Persistent Postorchiectomy Tumor Marker Elevation**

  These patients should be treated as having advanced stage disease. It is very important, however, to confirm the elevated AFP and beta-human chorionic gonadotropin (HCG) levels and also ensure there is not another reason for the elevation. Liver disease, marijuana use, and hypogonadism are all known causes of tumor marker elevation.

ADVANCED STAGE DISEASE

Advanced stage NSGCT includes all patients with persistent postorchiectomy tumor marker elevation. In addition to patients with stage IIC or stage III disease, advanced-stage disease also includes patients with an extragonadal primary (mediastinal or retroperitoneal). These patients all require induction chemotherapy. The primary choice of chemotherapy depends upon the IGCCCG risk classification.

- **Good-Risk NSGCT**

  This group includes patients with stage IS, IIA and IIB with persistent tumor marker elevation, IIC, or IIIA disease. Recommended chemotherapy includes four cycles of EP or three cycles of BEP. Randomized trials have shown both regimens to be generally well tolerated, with about 90% cure rate (8).

- **Intermediate-Risk NSGCT (Stage IIIB)**

  An additional cycle of BEP (four cycles) is considered standard of care. The expected cure rate is approximately 70% with this regimen (9).

- **Poor-Risk NSGCT (Stage IIIC)**

  Standard chemotherapy remains four cycles of BEP. However, the failure rate is high, so clinical trials are preferred if available. Etoposide/ifosfamide/cisplatin (VIP) has been compared to BEP and was found to be more toxic but equally effective (10). That being said, VIP remains a good option for patients who cannot tolerate bleomycin.

  Following induction chemotherapy, repeat CT scans in addition to serum tumor markers are required. If there is a complete response with normalization of the tumor markers, the patient is managed based on the original stage of the disease (surveillance vs. RPLND). If there is a partial response or a residual mass is present, the remaining site(s) of disease should be resected. Further treatment depends upon the histology of the resected lesions. If teratoma or necrosis is seen, no chemotherapy is needed, but if residual embryonal, yolk sac, choriocarcinoma, or seminoma element is identified, two cycles of chemotherapy (EP, VIP, vinblastine/ifosfamide/cisplatin [VeIP], or paclitaxel/ifosfamide/cisplatin [TIP]) are recommended (5).

  Patients with brain metastases at initial diagnosis have a poorer prognosis. Treatment of systemic disease is usually a priority in these patients, so cisplatin-based chemotherapy is usually given first. Residual disease can then be treated with radiation therapy (XRT) or surgery (5).

RELAPSED/REFRACTORY DISEASE

In patients who fail to respond to initial treatment or experience relapse, participation in clinical trials is encouraged (Table 30.1). Standard options include conventional dose chemotherapy (VeIP or TIP) or high-dose chemotherapy (carboplatin/etoposide [CE] or paclitaxel/ifosfamide/carboplatin/etoposide [TI-CE]) followed by autologous stem cell transplant. The TIGER trial is an ongoing phase 3 clinical trial that will hopefully answer which one of these options is clinically superior (Table 30.1).

Table 30.1 Currently Recruiting* Phase 2 and 3 Clinical Trials for Patients With Relapsed/Refractory NSGCT

Phase	Intervention/treatment	Primary outcome	Trial ID
3	TIGER trial: Paclitaxel, ifosfamide, and cisplatin (TIP) vs. HD chemotherapy with paclitaxel, ifosfamide, carboplatin, and etoposide (TICE) followed by ASCT	Overall survival	NCT02375204
2	Pegfilgrastim, actinomycin D, methotrexate, paclitaxel, oxaliplatin	Objective response rate	NCT01782339
	High-dose gemcitabine, docetaxel, melphalan, and carboplatin with ASCT vs. high-dose ifosfamide, carboplatin, and etoposide with ASCT	2-y event-free survival	NCT00936936
	Brentuximab vedotin	Objective response	NCT02689219
	TICE with dose intensification	Complete response rate	NCT00864318
	Sirolimus + erlotinib	Progression free rate and toxicity	NCT01962896
	Tandem ASCT following non-cross resistant HD chemotherapy vs. single ASCT following HD chemotherapy	Overall survival	NCT00432094
	Bevacizumab + HD ifosfamide, carboplatin, and etoposide (ICE) with intensification	Response and toxicity	NCT01966913

(continued)

Table 30.1 Currently Recruiting* Phase 2 and 3 Clinical Trials for Patients With Relapsed/Refractory NSGCT (continued)			
Phase	Intervention/treatment	Primary outcome	Trial ID
	Olaparib	Overall response rate	NCT02533765
	Gemcitabine, carboplatin, and veliparib	Disease free progression	NCT02860819

ASCT, autologous stem cell transplant; HD, high-dose; ICE, ifosfamide, carboplatin, and etoposide; NSGCT, nonseminomatous germ cell tumors.
*Trials open and recruiting as of January 15, 2017.

Several prognostic factors in patients with relapsed or refractory disease have been identified (11). Complete response to first-line therapy, low postorchiectomy serum tumor markers, and low-volume disease are considered relatively good prognostic factors. VeIP or TIP is a standard chemotherapy option in this situation, although high-dose chemotherapy with stem cell transplant is also an accepted option (5).

Poor prognostic factors include incomplete response to or progression during initial therapy, high postorchiectomy serum tumor markers, high-volume disease, or an extragonadal primary. These patients should be referred for clinical trials if available, but high-dose chemotherapy followed by autologous stem cell transplant or standard-dose salvage chemotherapy (TIP or VeIP) are both acceptable. Palliative chemotherapy or salvage surgery is also an option in carefully selected patients (5).

Palliative chemotherapy or radiation should be considered for patients with persistent or recurrent disease. Palliative chemotherapy options include combinations of gemcitabine, paclitaxel, and oxaliplatin, or oral etoposide (5).

SURVEILLANCE

Surveillance following successful treatment of NSGCT is vital to detect early recurrence and initiate treatment. Typical surveillance includes regular history and physicals, serum tumor markers, CT abdomen/pelvis, and chest radiographs.

The NCCN provides detailed interval recommendations for these tests depending on the clinical or pathologic stage of the disease (5).

> **KEY POINTS**
>
> - Patients with elevated AFP levels are treated as if they have nonseminomatous germ cell tumors, regardless of histology at orchiectomy.
> - Sperm banking should be offered to all patients prior to chemotherapy or RPLND.
> - Tumor markers for staging purposes should be measured after orchiectomy, with sufficient time given for normalization based on marker half-life.
> - In patients with early stage disease and good-risk advanced disease, cure rates are 90% or higher.
> - Patients with intermediate- or high-risk advanced disease have cure rates of 70% or less.

REFERENCES

1. American Joint Committee on Cancer. Testis. In: Amin MB, Edge SB, Greene FL, et al., eds. AJCC Cancer Staging Manual, 8th ed. Chicago, IL: Springer, 2017:727-735.
2. International Germ Cell Consensus Classification: a prognostic factor-based staging system for metastatic germ cell cancers. International Germ Cell Cancer Collaborative Group. *J Clin Oncol.* 1997;15:594-603.
3. Groll RJ, Warde P, Jewett MA. A comprehensive systematic review of testicular germ cell tumor surveillance. *Crit Rev Oncol Hematol.* 2007;64:182-197.
4. Kollmannsberger C, Tandstad T, Bedard PL, et al. Patterns of relapse in patients with clinical stage I testicular cancer managed with active surveillance. *J Clin Oncol.* 2015;33(1):51-57.
5. Motzer RJ, Jonasch E, Agarwal N, et al. National Comprehensive Cancer Network Practice Guidelines in Oncology: Testicular Cancer, National Comprehensive Cancer Network. Version 2.2016. Rockledge, PA; 2016.
6. Albers P, Siener R, Krege S, et al. Randomized phase III trial comparing retroperitoneal lymph node dissection with one course of bleomycin and etoposide plus cisplatin chemotherapy in the

adjuvant treatment of clinical stage I nonseminomatous testicular germ cell tumors: AUO trial AH 01/94 by the German Testicular Cancer Study Group. *J Clin Oncol.* 2008;26:2966-2972.

7. Weissbach L, Bussar-Maatz R, Flechtner H, et al. RPLND or primary chemotherapy in clinical stage IIA/B nonseminomatous germ cell tumors? Results of a prospective multicenter trial including quality of life assessment. *Eur Urol* 2000;37:582-594.

8. Jones RH, Vasey PA. Part II: testicular cancer—management of advanced disease. *Lancet Oncol.* 2003;4:738-747.

9. de Wit R, Stoter G, Sleijfer DT, et al. Four cycles of BEP vs. four cycles of VIP in patients with intermediate-prognosis metastatic testicular non-seminoma: a randomized study of the EORTC Genitourinary Tract Cancer Cooperative Group. European Organization for Research and Treatment of Cancer. *Br J Cancer.* 1998;78:828-832.

10. Nichols CR, Catalano PJ, Crawford ED, et al. Randomized comparison of cisplatin and etoposide and either bleomycin or ifosfamide in treatment of advanced disseminated germ cell tumors: an Eastern Cooperative Oncology Group, Southwest Oncology Group, and Cancer and Leukemia Group B Study. *J Clin Oncol.* 1998;16:1287-1293.

11. Lorch A, Beyer J, Bascoul-Mollevi C, et al. Prognostic factors in patients with metastatic germ cell tumors who experienced treatment failure with cisplatin-based first-line chemotherapy. *J Clin Oncol.* 2010;28:4906-4911.

Reproductive Considerations and Long-Term Complications of Therapy 31

Thiri Khin and Martha Pritchett Mims

INTRODUCTION

Testicular cancer accounts for 1% of all cancers in men and is the most common cancer in men between the ages of 15 and 35. Ninety-five percent of testicular carcinoma is germ cell tumor that can further be divided into seminoma and non-seminomatous germ cell tumor. Testicular carcinoma is one of the most curable cancers and with advances in treatment the overall survival is beyond 10 years in more than 95% of patients. Treatment of testicular cancer is multimodal with radical inguinal orchiectomy followed by surveillance versus chemotherapy and/or radiation therapy (RT) depending on the cancer stage. Given that the majority of patients are young and the cure rate is high, survivors of testicular cancer are faced with challenges of long-term adverse effects of various modalities of treatment.

REPRODUCTIVE CHALLENGES IN TESTICULAR CANCER

Infertility is a major concern since testicular cancer affects men in their reproductive years. Testicular cancer patients are at high risk for infertility and hypogonadism even before the treatment is started due to endocrine and metabolic effects of cancer, autoimmune effects, dysgonadogenesis, and congenital malformation of the testis such as cryptorchidism and hypospadias (1).

INTRINSIC EFFECTS OF TESTICULAR CANCER ON FERTILITY

Multiple studies have shown that more than 30% of testicular cancer patients have azoospermia or oligospermia prior to undergoing orchiectomy, and 50% have decreased sperm motility (2). Systemic effects of cancer such as fever and cytokine production can affect spermatogenesis. Cytokines also disturb normal endocrine pathways including the hypothalamic-pituitary-gonadal axis (3). In addition, hormone-producing testicular tumors affect spermatogenesis and cause changes in sex hormones. De Bruin et al have reported that patients with beta human chorionic gonadotropin (HCG)–producing testicular cancers have higher testosterone and estradiol, and lower follicle stimulating hormone (FSH), luteinizing hormone (LH), and sperm counts (4).

EFFECTS OF CANCER TREATMENT ON FERTILITY

The testis is highly susceptible to the toxic effects of radiation and chemotherapy since spermatogenesis involves rapid cell division. Cytotoxic chemotherapy and radiotherapy may produce long-lasting or persistent damage to primordial sperm cells, leading to oligo- or azoospermia. The risk of infertility is dependent on pubertal status at the start of treatment, the type of treatment used, the chemotherapy agent(s) administered, and number of cycles given. Men treated with chemotherapy and those treated with extended-field RT are at the highest risk. Standard treatment of advanced testicular cancer includes combination chemotherapy with cisplatin, bleomycin, and etoposide. A large European study involving 1,433 patients demonstrated that patients who received high-dose cisplatin (total dose >850 mg) had the lowest incidence of successful conception (38%) compared to surveillance (81%), low-dose cisplatin (62%), RT (61%), and retroperitoneal lymph node dissection (RPLND) (77%) (5). The type of surgery patients receive can also affect fertility and sexual dysfunction. Nonnerve sparing RPLND has the highest risk of sexual dysfunction, retrograde ejaculation, and anejaculation. Patients with dry ejaculation after treatment are the least likely to conceive. In addition, 0.6% of testicular cancer patients have synchronous tumors on the contralateral side and require bilateral orchiectomy. Psychosocial effects of cancer itself and treatment and anxiety also further diminish the chances of successful conception.

FERTILITY PRESERVATION

In light of the significant infertility risk in testicular cancer patients, discussion of infertility risk and methods of fertility preservation should be routinely incorporated in their care. Semen cryopreservation is considered the standard practice, and referral to a fertility specialist should be made before starting any treatment. If possible, baseline sperm count and sperm banking should be performed prior to the radiographic diagnostic evaluation in order to avoid radiation exposure of the sperm. Improvements in assisted reproductive techniques and cryopreservation have increased fertility rates; however, fewer than 30% of patients utilize sperm banking and testing before starting treatment. Reports show less than 10% proceed to conception with cryopreserved sperm. (6) Barriers to fertility preservation include lack of financial support, lack of proper knowledge of risks and benefits, lack of desire, and fear of delaying treatments. Despite multiple challenges hindering fertility and low use of fertility preservation methods, approximately 50% of testicular patients recover spermatogenesis in 2 years and 80% after 5 years. Cumulative posttreatment paternity rate is about 71% in a large European cohort described earlier (5).

TREATMENT-RELATED ADVERSE EFFECTS AND LONG-TERM COMPLICATIONS OF THERAPY

In addition to fertility challenges, testicular cancer survivors are at a higher risk of developing complications in multiple organs and systems following multimodality treatment.

Cardiovascular

Compared to the general population, testicular cancer survivors are not only at high risk of developing unfavorable cardiovascular risk factors such as metabolic syndrome, but also at higher risk of developing cardiovascular events such as coronary artery disease and thromboembolism. Factors associated with highest risk include mediastinal radiation and combination chemotherapy with cisplatin. The etiology of metabolic syndrome in testicular cancer is unclear.

Pulmonary

Bleomycin is an integral part of testicular cancer treatment. In a cohort of 835 patients, bleomycin-induced pulmonary toxicity was seen in 7% and 1% died as a result (7). Short-term bleomycin-induced pulmonary toxicity occurs in up to 46% of patients within 3 years of treatment and is usually mild and self-limited. A small number of patients develop long-term complications such as pulmonary fibrosis with mortality up to 10%. Patients who are treated with bleomycin are at risk of provoking pulmonary toxicity and respiratory failure when exposed to high oxygen levels in general anesthesia. Thus, it is important to educate patients and alert health care personnel of prior bleomycin use to avoid high oxygen concentration if possible. High cumulative dose of cisplatin has also been associated with restrictive lung disease in long-term survivors.

Renal

Renal dysfunction is seen during active treatment with cisplatin, and hydration is of utmost importance. In a prospective study following 85 patients over 14 years, the incidence of long-term renal dysfunction is seen in 29% of patients treated with multiagent chemotherapy (8).

Nervous System

Patients treated with cisplatin are at risk of developing peripheral neuropathy and ototoxicity. Neuropathy may persist for up to a decade after treatment. Cisplatin-induced ototoxicity manifests as hearing impairment, tinnitus, and high-frequency hearing loss.

Others

Patients treated with RT are at increased risk of late gastric and duodenal ulcers. Decreased bone mineral density and osteoporosis are also seen as a result of hypogonadism and late complications of chemotherapy and RT.

RISK OF SECONDARY MALIGNANCY

Testicular cancer survivors are more likely to develop second malignancies when compared to the general population. In the largest study to date, including 40,576 patients, there was an increased risk of solid cancers in men treated with RT (relative risk [RR] = 2), chemotherapy (RR =1.8), and with combined radiation and chemotherapy (RR = 2.9) (9). The most common second malignancies included lung, colon, bladder, pancreas, and stomach, which account for 60% of all solid tumors (9). Patients treated with combined chemotherapy are at increased risk of developing leukemia, but the incidence is less than 0.5%. Etoposide is a topoisomerase II inhibitor and is known to cause characteristic myeloid malignancy/leukemia involving chromosome translocation 11q23, and typically occurs within 1 to 3 years following treatment.

RISK OF RADIATION EXPOSURE

Testicular cancer patients are exposed to numerous imaging studies throughout the course of the disease and for many years thereafter for surveillance. Increased exposure to radiation has raised concerns over contributing to secondary malignancy. A Canadian study observed 2,569 testicular cancer patients over a median follow-up of 11 years. The median number of CT scans in the first 5 years was 10, and 14 patients developed secondary malignancy in this cohort. Radiation exposure was not associated with increased risk of secondary malignancy with hazard ratio (HR) 0.99 (95% confidence interval [CI] 0.95–1.04) (10). However, follow-up in this study was short and limited. Clinicians should always take into consideration a patient's age and the risk of excessive radiation in young survivors when planning for imaging.

KEY POINTS

- Both the cancer itself and its treatment affect fertility in testicular cancer patients.
- Age at diagnosis, type of surgery, and cumulative high dose of cisplatin are important predictors of successful conception in testicular cancer patients.
- Reproductive counseling and fertility preservation methods should be offered to all testicular cancer patients prior to starting treatment with RPLND or chemotherapy.
- Significant bleomycin toxicity can occur after exposure to high concentrations of oxygen; thus, testicular cancer survivors and the physicians caring for them should be aware of the risks following treatment.
- Treatment-related damage to the nervous system, the heart, and the kidneys should be monitored both during treatment and during long-term follow-up.
- RT and chemotherapy increase the risk of developing a secondary malignancy up to 2-fold in testicular cancer patients.

REFERENCES

1. Ostrowski KA, Walsh TJ. Infertility with testicular cancer. *Urol Clin North Am*. 2015;42(3):409-420.
2. Fosså SD, Abyholm T, Aakvaag A. Spermatogenesis and hormonal status after orchiectomy for cancer and before supplementary treatment. *Eur Urol*. 1984;10(3):173-177.
3. Nuver J, Smit AJ, Wolffenbuttel BH, et al. The metabolic syndrome and disturbances in hormone levels in long-term survivors of disseminated testicular cancer. *J Clin Oncol*. 2005;23(16):3718-3725.
4. De Bruin D, de Jong IJ, Arts EG, et al. Semen quality in men with disseminated testicular cancer: relation with human chorionic gonadotropin beta-subunit and pituitary gonadal hormones. *Fertil Steril*. 2009;91(6):2481-2486.
5. Brydøy M, Fosså SD, Klepp O, et al. Paternity following treatment for testicular cancer. *J Natl Cancer Inst*. 2005;97(21):1580-1588.
6. Girasole CR, Cookson MS, Smith JA Jr, et al. Sperm banking: use and outcomes in patients treated for testicular cancer. *BJU Int*. 2007;99(1):33-36.

7. O'Sullivan JM, Huddart RA, Norman AR, et al. Predicting the risk of bleomycin lung toxicity in patients with germ-cell tumours. *Ann Oncol*. 2003;14(1):91-96.
8. Fosså SD, Aass N, Winderen M, et al. Long-term renal function after treatment for malignant germ-cell tumors. *Ann Oncol*. 2002;13(2):222-228.
9. Travis LB, Fosså SD Schonfeld SJ, et al. Second cancers among 40,576 testicular cancer patients: focus on long-term survivors. *J Natl Cancer Inst*. 2005;97(18):1354-1365.
10. Van Walraven C, Fergusson D, Earle C, et al. Association of diagnostic radiation exposure and second abdominal-pelvic malignancies after testicular cancer. *J Clin Oncol*. 2011;29(21):2883-2888.

Controversies in the Management of Testicular Cancer 32

Ghana Kang and Martha Pritchett Mims

INTRODUCTION

While many aspects of the care of testicular cancer patients and survivors are established, there are a number of areas in which controversy continues to exist. A few of these areas are described next.

Case 1: A 33-year-old man was treated with bleomycin, etoposide, and cisplatin (BEP) for a clinical stage IIA nonseminomatous germ cell tumor (NSGCT). A restaging CT scan showed residual retroperitoneal lymph nodes measuring up to 0.9 cm.

Question 1: Is postchemotherapy retroperitoneal lymph node dissection (RPLND) for patients with sub-centimeter residual masses indicated?

Standards defining the size of "normal" retroperitoneal lymph nodes differ depending on the institution; thus, the indication for RPLND following chemotherapy is controversial (1). Ehrlich et al reported on 141 patients who underwent chemotherapy for metastatic NSGCTs with radiographic complete response (defined as residual mass <1 cm) and subsequent management with surveillance (2). After a median follow-up of 15.5 years, only 12 experienced relapse, and of these only four died. Interestingly, five patients relapsed after more than 2 years (range 3–13 years), emphasizing the need for long-term surveillance in testicular cancer patients. The authors concluded that relapses are rare and potentially curable with treatment on relapse. However, other investigators have identified viable germ cell tumor (GCT) or teratoma in patients with subcentimeter retroperitoneal adenopathy. Steyerberg et al evaluated small retroperitoneal masses and found teratoma or viable GCT in 45% of lesions measuring 1.1 mm to 2.0 cm and in 28% of lesions measuring up to 1.0 cm on CT imaging (3). These numbers are concerning since unresected GCTs are likely to relapse and more likely to be resistant to chemotherapy. Growing teratomas may be more difficult to resect than immediately after chemotherapy, and a risk of malignant transformation has been reported. As a result of this information, some institutions advocate postchemotherapy RPLND in select patients with radiographically detectable retroperitoneal masses after chemotherapy.

Question 2: This patient is now considering RPLND, but he is extremely concerned about the risk of retrograde ejaculation after the operation. What are the advantages and concerns of contemporary retroperitoneal lymph node dissection techniques?

The role of RPLND is well established in the management of GCT; however, the extent of resection remains an area of controversy. Before effective chemotherapy was available, extensive resection and removal of all lymph nodes in the retroperitoneum was emphasized. Later studies demonstrated that resection of nodes above the renal hilum provided no additional benefit, but did increase morbidity in patients with low-stage disease. More recently, the focus on preservation of sympathetic innervation to prevent retrograde ejaculation and infertility, which led to the development of nerve-sparing bilateral template RPLND. In high-volume centers, this approach has resulted in antegrade ejaculation in more than 95% of patients undergoing primary RPLND. Anatomic mapping studies led to the development of modified unilateral RPLND, whose goal is to minimize resection while maintaining cancer control (4). The major concern for this approach is the danger of unresected disease outside the resection template, and the primary criticism of these mapping studies was their retrospective nature. Two studies from the Memorial Sloan-Kettering group evaluated the incidence of disease outside the resection template in patients undergoing both primary and postchemotherapy RPLND (5,6). Depending on the setting, up to 32% of patients had either viable GCT or teratoma outside the resection template. These studies challenge the equivalence of bilateral and unilateral modified template RPLND, and thus the role of modified unilateral RPLND remains controversial.

Case 2: A 46-year-old man with a history of heavy smoking who was recently diagnosed with stage IIB NSGCT is in your office to discuss options for chemotherapy.

Question 3: Is BEP equivalent to etoposide/cisplatin (EP)?
Cisplatin combination therapy cures even advanced GCTs, and several large studies have demonstrated that carboplatin is inferior to cisplatin for achieving cure (7). Standard chemotherapy treatments have not changed since BEP became a standard regimen for GCTs. The value of using bleomycin with its increased risk of pulmonary toxicity has been questioned in several studies. The Australasian Germ Cell Trial Group compared PVB (cisplatin/vinblastine/bleomycin) with PV (cisplatin/vinblastine) and concluded that there were an increased number of cancer deaths in the PV arm. Thirty-four percent of patients in the PVB arm experienced pulmonary toxicity, but the authors felt that the difference in survival far outweighed the lung issues. In a study conducted by the Genito-Urinary Group of the French Federation of Cancer Centers (GETUG), 270 patients with NSGCT were randomized to receive either three cycles of BEP or four cycles of EP. The 4-year event-free survival rates were 91% for the BEP group and 86% for the EP group ($P = .135$) (8). The 4-year overall survival rates were not significantly different (5 deaths vs. 12 deaths, respectively [$P = .096$]). Although outcome did not reach statistical significance, bleomycin has maintained its important role in curative treatment. Most oncologists reserve EP for those who have contraindication to the use of bleomycin. In making a choice between regimens, one must weigh the toxicities associated with the increased cumulative dose of cisplatin and etoposide in four cycles of EP against the risk of pulmonary toxicity from bleomycin in three cycles of BEP. The GETUG demonstrated more neurotoxicity, dermatitis, and Raynaud phenomenon in patients receiving BEP and more high-grade neutropenia in those receiving EP. There was no statistically significant difference in neutropenic fever and pulmonary toxicity between the two arms.

Question 4: This patient successfully completed his chemotherapy with BEP with no evidence of disease, but has not been compliant with surveillance. He now developed shortness of breath 2 years after completion of chemotherapy and was found to have multiple lung masses bilaterally. The biopsy confirmed recurrent NSGCT. What are the options for second-line chemotherapy?

Overall, 20% to 30% of patients presenting with metastatic GCT are refractory to treatment or relapse after initial chemotherapy. Few prospective studies have addressed the issue of optimal treatment in this setting, and no studies gave compared salvage chemotherapy with high-dose chemotherapy with stem cell rescue. Since the advent of BEP as the optimal initial regimen for GCT, etoposide is generally not used in second-line therapy. Combinations of ifosfamide and cisplatin with either vinblastine (VeIP) or paclitaxel (TIP) are typically used in this setting. The largest single study of VeIP in the second line following EP or BEP in the first line demonstrated 49.6% disease-free status after four cycles of treatment and/or surgical resection of residual disease (9). Seven-year survival in the VeIP study was 32%. The largest study of TIP in the second line in patients who had received BEP was conducted by the British Medical Research Council. The complete response (CR) rate in the study was 31%, with a 1-year failure-free survival of 38% (10). Patients with primary mediastinal GCTs and late relapse were included in this study as they were in the large VeIP study. Comparison of VeIP and TIP in the second line was undertaken in a randomized phase 3 study, but the study was stopped due to poor accrual leaving the choice of regimen in this setting open.

There are also data examining high-dose chemotherapy (HDCT) with stem cell rescue in the second-line setting. The IT-94 study, a European multicenter study, randomized patients who failed first-line platinum containing regimens to either four cycles of VIP or VeIP versus three cycles of VeIP/VIP followed by HDCT with carboplatin, etoposide, and cyclophosphamide with stem cell rescue (11). CR rates were similar in both arms and there was no survival benefit to HDCT, although the study has been criticized for the fact that only one cycle of HDCT was given, and only 81% of patients in the HDCT arm proceeded to transplant. Retrospective data from nearly 2,000 patients treated with conventional chemotherapy and HDCT demonstrated superior progression free survival and overall survival in all risk categories (12). Patients with favorable prognostic features may achieve durable remissions without HDCT and its attendant risks. However, the criteria for optimal patient selection remain unclear, and many centers employ a risk stratification algorithm to assist in advising patients. The Alliance randomized phase 3 trial of initial salvage chemotherapy for patients with germ cell tumors (NCT02375204), which compares survival outcomes with TIP versus paclitaxel/ifosfamide/carboplatin/etoposide (TI-CE) for relapsed or refractory GCT patients, should resolve this controversy.

KEY POINTS

- Standards for defining "normal"-sized retroperitoneal nodes after primary chemotherapy vary by institution, and normal size does not ensure that relapse will not occur.
- Resection templates for RPLND are controversial, with the most conservative approach being nerve sparing bilateral template resection.
- Most oncologists favor BEP for front-line therapy, reserving EP for those with contraindication to bleomycin.
- Second-line chemotherapy for refractory or relapsed disease should not include etoposide if that drug was used in the front-line setting.
- The value of HDCT with stem cell transplant over second-line chemotherapy has not yet been proven in a randomized controlled trial.

REFERENCES

1. Tarin T, Carver B, Sheinfeld J. The role of lymphadenectomy for testicular cancer: indications, controversies, and complications. *Urol Clin N Am*. 2011;38:439-449.
2. Ehrlich Y, Brames M, Beck S, et al. Long-term follow-up of cisplatin combination chemotherapy in patients with disseminated nonseminomatous germ cell tumors: is a post-chemotherapy

retroperitoneal lymph node dissection needed after complete remission? *J Clin Oncol*. 2010;28:531-536.
3. Steyerberg EW, Keizer HJ, Fossa SD, et al. Prediction of residual retroperitoneal mass histology after chemotherapy for metastatic nonseminomatous germ cell tumor: multivariate analysis of individual patient data from six study groups. *J Clin Oncol*. 1995;13:1177-1187.
4. Katz M, Eggener S. The evolution, controversies, and potential pitfalls of modified retroperitoneal lymph node dissection templates. *World J Urol*. 2009;27:477-483.
5. Eggener SE, Carver BS, Sharp DS, et al. Incidence of disease outside modified retroperitoneal lymph node dissection templates in clinical stage I or IIA nonseminomatous germ cell testicular cancer. *J Urol*. 2007;177:937-942.
6. Carver BS, Shayegan B, Eggener S, et al. Incidence of metastatic nonseminomatous germ cell tumor outside the boundaries of a modified postchemotherapy retroperitoneal lymph node dissection. *J Clin Oncol*. 2007;25:4365-4369.
7. In G, Dorff T. Chemotherapy for good-risk nonseminomatous germ cell tumors current concepts and controversies. *Urol Clin N Am*. 2015;42:347-357.
8. Culine S, Kerbrat P, Kramar A, et al. Refining the optimal chemotherapy regimen for good-risk metastatic nonseminomatous germ-cell tumors: a randomized trial of the Genito-Urinary Group of the French Federation of Cancer Centers (GETUG T93BP). *Ann Oncol*. 2007;18:917-924.
9. Loehrer PJ, Gonin R, Nichols CR, et al. Vinblastine plus ifosfamide plus cisplatin as initial salvage therapy in recurrent germ cell tumor. *J Clin Oncol*. 1998;16:2500-2504.
10. Mead GM, Cullen MH, Huddart R, et al. A phase II trial of TIP (paclitaxel, ifosfamide and cisplatin) given as second-line (post-BEP) salvage chemotherapy for patients with metastatic germ cell cancer: a medical research council trial. *Br J Cancer*. 2005;93:178-184.
11. Pico JL, Rosti G, Kramar A, et al. A randomised trial of high-dose chemotherapy in the salvage treatment of patients failing first-line platinum chemotherapy for advanced germ cell tumours. *Ann Oncol*. 2005;16:1152-1159.
12. Lorch A, Beyer J, Bascoul-Mollevi C, et al. Prognostic factors in patients with metastatic germ cell tumors who experienced treatment failure with cisplatin-based first-line chemotherapy. *J Clin Oncol*. 2010; 28:4906-4911.

PENILE CANCER

Treatment of Early Stage Penile Cancer 33

Guilherme Godoy

INTRODUCTION

Penile cancer is a rare malignancy that involves the squamous mucosal epithelia of the glans, coronal sulcus, and inner prepuce, potentially extending to the corpora, urethra, and penile shaft in more advanced stages. Tumors arising from the mid and proximal penile shaft skin are extremely uncommon.

It affects men in their fifties, with peak incidence between the ages of 50 and 70 years. Cancer of the penis is associated with significant morbidity and mortality with important impact in both sexual and urinary functions and potentially devastating psychologic consequences to the patients (1,2).

The overall 5-year cancer-specific survival is approximately 50%, ranging from 85% to 29%-40% in those without and with lymph node metastasis, respectively, down to <10% in those with pelvic lymph node involvement (3,4).

It represents 0.4% to 0.6% of all malignant tumors among men in the United States and Europe, with an average reported incidence of 1:100,000 men per year in the United States (2,5). In 2017, 2,120 new cases are estimated, with 360 expected deaths from this disease in the United States (6). The incidence is variable according to the geographical region. The highest rates are in some developing countries of Asia, Africa, and South America, where penile cancer comprises up to 20% of all malignancies (7).

The most common histological type is the conventional squamous cell carcinoma (SCC), which comprises approximately 95% of all penile cancers, but several other morphological subtypes and variants exist. Table 33.1 illustrates the

Table 33.1 Histopathologic Subtypes of Penile Carcinoma

	Subtype	Prognosis
Common subtypes	Common SCC	variable*
	Warty carcinoma	good
	Verrucous carcinoma	good
	Papillary carcinoma	good
	Wartybasaloid carcinoma	poor
	Basaloid carcinoma	poor
	Sarcomatoid carcinoma	very poor
	Mixed carcinoma	variable
Rare subtypes	Pseudohyperplastic carcinoma	good
	Carcinoma cuniculatum	good
	Adenosquamous carcinoma	intermediate
	Pseudoglandular carcinoma	poor
	Mucoepidermoid carcinoma	poor
	Clear cell variant	poor

SCC, squamous-cell carcinoma.

*Depends on stage/grade and presence of other risk factors.

Source: Adapted from Ref. (8). Pizzocaro G, Algaba F, Horenblas S, et al. EAU penile cancer guidelines 2009. *Eur Urol*. 2010;57(6):1002–1012.

variable histopathological presentations of these lesions with their respective prognosis (8).

Several premalignant lesions are also recognized. Appropriate diagnosis and treatment of these lesions are important to prevent the development of invasive tumor stages. Table 33.2 illustrates the main described premalignant lesions (8).

The primary lesion follows a progressive and local pattern of growth and infiltration in the penis, invading deeply from the skin to the corpora and urethra. Metastatic spread occurs predominantly via lymphatic dissemination in a stepwise fashion, starting from the superficial to the deep inguinal lymph nodes before reaching the pelvic lymph nodes and other organs. Therefore, early diagnosis and treatment are key to successful management of the disease.

Although surgical excision is the mainstay of the treatment of the early forms of the disease, a multimodal approach with the

Table 33.2 Premalignant Lesions Associated With Penile Carcinoma	
Sporadically associated	Cutaneous horn
	Bowenoid papulosis
	Lichen sclerosus (balanitis xerotic obliterans)
Premalignant lesions*	Penile intraepithelial neoplasia grade III (PIN or PeIN)
	Giant condylomata (Buschke-Löwenstein disease)
	Erythroplasia of Queyrat
	Bowen's disease
	Paget's disease

*Up to a third transform into invasive cancer.

Source: Adapted from Ref. (8). Pizzocaro G, Algaba F, Horenblas S, et al. EAU penile cancer guidelines 2009. *Eur Urol*. 2010;57(6):1002-1012.

integration of radiation and chemotherapy is critical to appropriate management of more advanced stages of this disease.

RISK FACTORS

The presence of **phimosis and uncircumcised foreskin** is an important and very well described risk factor associated with the development of penile cancer. The lifetime risk of developing penile cancer in uncircumcised American men is estimated to be 1:400, compared to 1:100,000 in circumcised men. Especially when performed in the prepubertal phase, there is a 22-fold risk reduction associated with circumcision. The benefit in penile cancer prevention seems to be maximized when it is performed in the neonatal period. In countries where most circumcisions are performed in newborns, the reported incidence rates are lower than 0.1:100,000 men (9). Furthermore, among 50,000 cases and 10,000 deaths from penile cancer occurring between 1930 and 1990, only 10 were documented in circumcised patients, all of whom underwent circumcision after puberty (10).

Other important described risk factors that are associated with the presence of phimosis or uncircumcised foreskin in most cases are **balanitis, balanoposthitis, chronic** inflammatory conditions (lichen sclerosus or balanitis xerotica obliterans), poor genital hygiene (accumulation of smegma), and lower socioeconomic status.

The history of sexually transmitted diseases, especially **HIV and human papillomavirus (HPV) infection**, is also an important risk factor. In general, the majority (up to 80%) of penile cancers are related to HPV infection, specifically the serotypes 16 and 18 (highest association), and also 31, 33 and other serotypes (1,2,11–13).

Uncircumcised men have a 5 to 10 times higher chance of acquiring HPV infection. This association is probably the most important association of factors (uncircumcised foreskin and HPV infection) for the development of the disease. HIV infection has also been reported to increase the risk of penile cancer by 8 fold (14).

Other risk factors include **cigarette smoking**, which is reported to increase the risk of developing penile cancer by 3 to 4.5 times, and the exposure to **psoralen plus ultraviolet A radiation**, a form of photochemotherapy used for the treatment of a variety of skin conditions, including psoriasis, vitiligo, and eczema.

DIAGNOSIS AND STAGING

The most common presentation is the presence of a sessile and painless penile tumor involving the glans and/or inner prepuce, or a palpable mass underlying the uncircumcised foreskin.

It can be associated with pain, discharge, bleeding, and foul odor, if secondarily infected or with presence of necrotic areas in more advanced lesions. At later stages, patients can present with palpable or ulcerated inguinal nodal metastasis and even constitutional symptoms.

The lesion itself can be characterized as nodular, ulcerative, or fungating. However, early stages may be more subtle, presenting just as discoloration, plaques, or small skin ulcers. Any lesion that does not heal after a short period of monitoring for 2 to 3 weeks with proper hygiene and skin care should be biopsied.

Tables 33.1 and 33.2 list the different types of histologic variations and the recognized premalignant lesions, also known as penile intraepithelial neoplasia (PeIN), illustrating the different possible presenting forms of the disease.

Biopsy is the mainstay of histopathological diagnosis. Its extent should take into consideration the location of the lesion and assess depth of invasion for staging purposes. The biopsy will also inform important risk factors, such as the histologic subtype, presence of lymph vascular invasion, and the degree of cell anaplasia (classifying the tumors according to their differentiation status).

In small and superficial lesions, an excisional biopsy may be both diagnostic and therapeutic. Tumors confined to the prepuce are perfect examples of such lesions that can be managed with a circumcision.

Physical exam of the bilateral inguinal lymph nodes is critical for proper staging. The use of ultrasonography and axial imaging (CT or MRI) may aid in further characterization and staging of both the primary tumor and inguinal lymph nodes. Information such as number of involved lymph nodes, location, size, and mobility are meaningful for decision-making. These need to be assessed bilaterally at presentation and at every visit during follow-up in those cases under surveillance. Complete staging for invasive tumors should also include imaging of the chest, abdomen, and pelvis (usually starting with a chest x-ray and CT of abdomen and pelvis).

Recently, the use of positron emission tomography scan (PET) with CT scan has been very useful in the diagnosis of regional metastatic disease (15,16).

The staging system most commonly used in penile cancer is the American Joint Commission on Cancer (AJCC) tumor, node, and metastasis (TNM) system (Table 33.3) (17).

Table 33.3 Penile Carcinoma TNM Staging System

Primary Tumor (T)	
TX	Primary tumor cannot be assessed
T0	No evidence of primary tumor
Ta	Noninvasive localized squamous cell carcinoma
Tis	Carcinoma in situ (Penile intraepithelial neoplasm [PeIn])
T1a	Tumor invades subepithelial connective tissue without lymph vascular or perineural invasion and is not poorly differentiated

(continued)

Table 33.3 Penile Carcinoma TNM Staging System (*continued*)	
T1b	Tumor invades subepithelial connective tissue with lymph vascular or perineural invasion or is poorly differentiated
T2	Tumor invades corpus spongiosum with or without urethral invasion
T3	Tumor invades corpora cavernosum with or without urethral invasion
T4	Tumor invades into adjacent structures (i.e., scrotum, prostate, pubic bone)
Regional Lymph Nodes (N)	
cNX	Regional lymph nodes cannot be assessed
pNX	Lymph node metastasis cannot be assessed.
cN0	No palpable or visibly enlarged lymph node metastasis
pN0	No lymph node metastasis
cN1	Palpable mobile unilateral inguinal lymph node
pN1	Metastasis in ≤2 unilateral inguinal nodes, no extracapsular extension
cN2	Palpable mobile ≥2 unilateral or bilateral inguinal lymph node metastases
pN2	Metastasis in ≥3 unilateral or bilateral inguinal lymph node metastases
cN3	Palpable fixed inguinal nodal mass or pelvic lymphadenopathy unilateral or bilateral
pN3	Extranodal extension of lymph node metastasis or pelvic lymph node metastasis
Distant Metastasis (M)	
M0	No distant metastasis
M1	Distant metastasis

c, clinical assessment; p, pathologic assessment; TNM, tumor, node, and metastasis.

Source: Adapted from Ref. (17). American Joint Committee on Cancer. Penis. In: Amin MB, Edge SB, Greene FL, et al., eds. *AJCC Cancer Staging Manual*. 8th ed. Chicago, IL: Springer; 2017:701–714.

TREATMENT MODALITIES FOR THE PRIMARY LESION

The choice of treatment depends on the location, size, clinical stage and grade, but also on the surgeon's experience and the patient's desire to preserve as much as possible of function and cosmetics.

Topical treatments involve the use of agents that either destroy the tumor cells or stimulate the patient's immune system to do so. These include topical application of 5% 5-fluorouracil (5-FU) cream and 5% imiquimod cream. These strategies are mostly used for penile carcinoma in situ or verrucous non-invasive lesions (Tis or Ta).

Topical agents tend to be offered up front, with 5% 5-FU cream as first line therapy, followed by imiquimod as second line after recurrence. Complete response rates reported with these therapies range between 57% and 74% with a median follow-up of approximately 3 years (18,19). The treatment can be repeated in case of partial response with residual lesion, or limited recurrent disease.

In the lack of response to topical agents, the treatment should escalate to ablative or excisional approaches.

Ablation techniques involve mainly the use of laser (carbon dioxide [CO_2] or Neodymium:Yttrium-Aluminum-Garnet [Nd:YAG] with or without potassium titanyl phosphate [KTP]). Our personal preference is for the CO_2 laser because of the smaller depth of penetration, better control over the ablation area, and superior healing results. Peniscopy examination with 3% to 5% acetic acid application can be utilized to facilitate identification of subtle HPV lesions that become acetowhite. The laser ablation approach is recommended only in early stages of the disease such as Tis and select small Ta or T1G1-2 lesions. The ablated areas heal by secondary intention and have favorable cosmetic results after full re-epithelization. However, this procedure requires training in laser therapy and dedicated personal protection equipment such as a plume evacuator.

Circumcision is recommended for lesions localized and limited to the foreskin. It is not only diagnostic, but it is also surgically effective as a therapeutic option in some select non-invasive localized lesions.

Mohs micrographic surgery is utilized in select cases, where the extent of the resection needs to be as limited as possible while assuring negative margins, such as in the glans or the shaft of the penis. In this technique, normally performed by trained dermatologists, the lesion is mapped in a grid. Serial, very thin resections are taken and frozen analyzed to reach only the extent and depth necessary to achieve negative margins around the tumor.

The extent of **surgical resection** may vary from a total glansectomy in more distal tumors limited to the glans, to partial penectomy (partial amputation of the penis) in invasive but still distal tumors, to total penectomy with perineal urethrostomy in those tumors that are more bulky and/or extend more proximally in the penile shaft.

As a principle, any surgical resection should result in free frozen section margins and at the same time cause as minimal impact as possible to urinary and sexual function, with acceptable cosmetic results whenever possible. When using penile conservation techniques, resurfacing of the glans and utilization of various types of split- or full-thickness skin graft techniques may be required. Additionally, all penile conservation techniques require close and frequent postoperative follow-up to monitor tumor resection margins for possible local recurrence.

For partial penectomies, a minimal margin of 1 cm (formerly 2 cm) is considered safe and is currently recommended. However, confirmation with frozen sections during the case is still necessary to rule out microscopic involvement of the margins. As a general guideline, the residual penile stump should be long enough to allow the patient to void in an upright position without the need to push away the scrotum. Otherwise, a perineal urethrostomy should be created instead. Approximately two thirds of the patients retain sexual activity after a partial penectomy, so attention to the preservation of the longest penile stump possible is an important consideration with this technique (20).

Technically the surgical procedures are not complicated, but the consequences can be devastating from the psychological standpoint. Psychiatric preoperative evaluation and postoperative follow-up is recommended, especially in patients undergoing a total penectomy.

Brachytherapy and external beam radiation therapy (EBRT) can also be utilized in select cases with adequate control of the tumor and the added benefit of avoiding a surgical amputation of the penis. Depending on the stage, grade, size, and location of the lesion, there are opportunities for utilization of brachytherapy or EBRT with or without associated chemotherapy.

Brachytherapy can be considered after excisional biopsies or in recurrent tumors after wide local excisions, but should not be performed after total or partial penectomies. It is usually recommended for small lesions located in the glans (T1G3-4 and select T2). Tumor size <4 cm seems to be associated with better outcomes (21). EBRT with or without chemotherapy is reserved for larger and higher stage lesions, with consideration for prophylactic irradiation to the inguinal lymph nodes. Surgically unresectable tumors are best managed with chemoradiation protocols.

As a principle, circumcision should always be performed before any radiation therapy modality to prevent phimosis. Rigorous case selection and close monitoring after treatment are critical to achieve and maintain adequate oncological outcomes after radiation therapy.

Any radiation therapy modality for penile cancer should only be performed in centers of excellence and with experience in treating the disease.

MANAGEMENT OF THE REGIONAL LYMPH NODES

The management of regional lymph nodes in the inguinal areas and pelvis is an integral component of the treatment of penile cancer, as these are the main and first landing sites of metastatic spread from the SCC lesions.

The presence and extent of regional lymph node metastasis is the single most important prognostic factor associated with long-term survival of men with invasive penile cancer (22). Lymphatic spread in penile carcinoma happens in a sequential, progressive manner with tumor cells migrating first to superficial and deep inguinal chains before progressing to pelvic nodes. There are no reported cases of pelvic lymph node involvement without concomitant or previous involvement of the inguinal lymph nodes (skip metastasis) (23–29).

The incidence of enlarged and palpable lymph nodes in the groin associated with penile cancer at presentation is approximately 30% to 60%. Conversely, node metastases are diagnosed in up to 25% of cases with negative signs for inguinal lymphadenopathy (30).

The traditional approach to palpable inguinal nodes has been abandoned, where men were first treated with a course of antibiotics before the decision for the inguinal lymph node dissection. Currently these men are assessed with ultrasound-guided fine-needle aspiration and/or excisional nodal biopsy for confirmation. In more advanced stages, the recommendation for bilateral inguinal lymph node dissection is made based on the presence of risk factors in the primary tumor.

Surgical inguinal dissection during lymphadenectomy is potentially associated with significant morbidity, including skin flap necrosis, lymphocele, cellulitis, and lower extremity lymphedema. In order to minimize or prevent these complications, new strategies were developed to avoid unnecessary inguinal exploration in clinically negative groins and low-risk patients. In addition, more limited and conservative templates of dissection were also proposed.

An Italian multicenter retrospective study generated a nomogram to estimate the probability of inguinal nodal metastasis. The main risk factors were the presence of lymph vascular invasion, palpable inguinal nodes, and invasive or poorly differentiated tumors (31). The presence of these features helps to stratify patients in risk groups and aids in the decision making about recommending inguinal lymph node dissections.

A modified or standard-template inguinal lymph node dissection is usually recommended for high-risk men with non-palpable nodes, as occult metastatic disease ranges from 68% to 73% (32–34). In patients with non-palpable inguinal nodes and the absence of high-risk primary tumor features for node metastasis, the groins can be safely observed or assessed with the dynamic sentinel lymph node biopsy (DSLNB) technique, when available.

The DSLNB procedure involves the injection of ^{99m}Tc colloid intradermally in the primary tumor, with next day identification of the sentinel lymph node for biopsy with both the gamma detection probe and also visually after injection of vital blue dye. Under this technique, inguinal lymph node dissection is only performed in those patients where the sentinel node biopsy reveals the presence of metastatic carcinoma. Recently, with the integration of preoperative inguinal ultrasound and fine-needle aspiration to the DSLNB technique, false-negative rates have improved from 19.2% to 4.8%, with the potential additional benefit that the modified technique may reduce the need for a bilateral groin dissection (35–37).

Because of the numerous details in the DSLNB procedures, it should only be recommended and performed if the treating physician has experience with the technique (28).

Modified surgical templates of dissection were also created to minimize morbidity of the resection by limiting the extent of the dissection. These surgical modifications include shorter skin incisions, limited extent of dissection focused on medial and superior aspects of femoral artery and fossa ovalis only, preservation of the saphenous vein, and elimination of the need for the use of a sartorius muscle transposition flap to cover exposed femoral vessels. In the presence of a positive inguinal lymph node in frozen sections, the dissection should be converted to a standard full-template inguinal lymphadenectomy.

In the absence of DSLNB availability, inguinal lymph node dissection should always be bilateral, as it is impossible to predict laterality of involvement in patients with high-risk primary tumors. Even with unilateral palpable disease, about 30% of cases have non-palpable nodal micrometastasis, therefore justifying a routine bilateral surgical approach (38).

Men with high-risk tumor features and clinically negative groins have better survival outcomes with immediate rather than with delayed inguinal lymph node dissection, supporting the potential therapeutic benefit of removing the sites of micrometastasis early. For those who refuse or are under surveillance for low-risk tumors, the expected median time to inguinal recurrence after treatment of the primary tumor is approximately 6 months, with the great majority (90%) occurring within 3 years and virtually all (100%) by 5 years of follow-up (25,29,34).

Patients with 2 or more pathologically positive inguinal nodes and/or with extranodal extension need a pelvic lymph node dissection in the same or in a separate surgical procedure. There is controversy about whether there is indication for bilateral pelvic lymph node dissection in the presence of unilateral inguinal nodal disease.

Men with only one positive inguinal lymph node, absence of extranodal extension, or high-grade disease have a risk of pelvic nodal metastasis of 5%. In this case the subsequent ipsilateral pelvic node dissection may be omitted (39). Conversely, in the presence of 4 or more positive nodes or extranodal extension, there is indication for bilateral pelvic lymph node dissection (40).

Patients with bulky inguinal lymphadenopathy (defined as the presence of a lymph node ≥ 4 cm, bilateral nodal disease, or fixed inguinal nodal masses) may benefit from neoadjuvant chemotherapy regimens to facilitate surgical procedure or to render fixed masses resectable.

Men who have an intermediate- or high-risk primary tumor treated with radiation therapy modalities should also consider having prophylactic radiation therapy applied to the inguinal regions in the absence of palpable disease.

CONCLUSION

Penile cancer is a rare, but potentially aggressive disease with profound impact in men's sexual, urinary, and psychologic functions. As the main histological subtype is SCC, the most important metastatic pathway is via lymphatic spread to bilateral inguinal and pelvic lymph nodes. Treatment of the regional lymph nodes is an integral component of the management of the disease.

Operative intervention is the mainstay in the management of both the primary lesion and the lymph node metastasis, serving diagnostic, therapeutic, and palliative roles. At early stages, the balance of care lies between conservative approaches with concerns to cosmetics and function, while minimizing morbidity and ensuring cancer control. In more advanced disease, more radical and extensive surgical procedures combined with a multimodal approach including radiation therapy and chemotherapy provide the best chance for cure.

Close follow-up and surveillance after treatment are critical, as local recurrences are not rare, systemic therapy efficacy is limited, and salvage surgical approaches are often curative for localized resectable disease.

KEY POINTS

- Squamous-cell carcinoma is the most common histological type.
- Surgical resection is the mainstay in the management of both the primary lesion and the lymph node metastasis, serving diagnostic, therapeutic, and palliative roles.
- The most important metastatic pathway is via lymphatic spread to bilateral inguinal and pelvic lymph nodes in a sequential and progressive manner.
- Treatment of the regional lymph nodes is an integral component of the management of the disease.
- In early tumor stages, organ- and function-preservation techniques can be utilized, while multimodal radical treatment approaches are needed to control more advanced stages of the disease.

REFERENCES

1. Pow-Sang MR, Ferreira U, Pow-Sang JM, et al. Epidemiology and natural history of penile cancer. *Urology*. 2010;76(2 Suppl 1):S2-S6.
2. Presti JC. Genital tumors. In: McAninch JW, Lue TF, eds. *Smith and Tanagho's General Urology*. 18th ed. New York, NY: McGraw-Hill/Lange; 2013.
3. Horenblas S. Lymphadenectomy for squamous cell carcinoma of the penis. Part 2: the role and technique of lymph node dissection. *BJU Int*. 2001;88(5):473-483.
4. Russo P, Horenblas S. Surgical Management of Penile Carcer. In: Scardino PT, Linehan WM, Zelefsky MJ, et al., eds. *Comprehensive Textbook of Genitourinary Oncology*. 4th ed. Baltimore, MD: Wolters Kluwer-Lippincott Williams & Wilkins; 2011:811-822.
5. Pettaway CA, Crook JM, Pagliaro LC. Penile carcinoma. In: Wein AJ, Kavoussi LR, Partin AW, et al., eds. *Campbell-Walsh Urology*. 10th ed. Philadelphia, PA: Elsevier; 2016:846-878.
6. Siegel RL, Miller KD, Jemal A. Cancer Statistics, 2017. *CA Cancer J Clin*. 2017;67(1):7-30.
7. Curado MP, Edwards B, Shin HR, et al. eds. *Cancer Incidence in Five Continents*. Vol IX. Lyon: IARC Scientific; 2007. http://www.iarc.fr/en/publications/pdfs-online/epi/sp160/CI15vol9.pdf. Accessed January 27, 2017.

8. Pizzocaro G, Algaba F, Horenblas S, et al. EAU penile cancer guidelines 2009. *Eur Urol*. 2010;57(6):1002-1012.
9. Schoen EJ. Neonatal circumcision and penile cancer. Evidence that circumcision is protective is overwhelming. *BMJ*. 1996;313(7048):46-47.
10. Schoen EJ. The relationship between circumcision and cancer of the penis. *CA Cancer J Clin*. 1991;41(5):306-309.
11. Daling JR, Madeleine MM, Johnson LG, et al. Penile cancer: importance of circumcision, human papillomavirus and smoking in in situ and invasive disease. *Int J Cancer*. 2005;116(4):606-616.
12. Dillner J, von Krogh G, Horenblas S, et al. Etiology of squamous cell carcinoma of the penis. *Scand J Urol Nephrol Suppl*. 2000:34189-34193.
13. Sarkar FH, Miles BJ, Plieth DH, et al. Detection of human papillomavirus in squamous neoplasm of the penis. *J Urol*. 1992;147(2):389-392.
14. Engels EA, Pfeiffer RM, Goedert JJ, et al. Trends in cancer risk among people with AIDS in the United States 1980–2002. *AIDS*. 2006;20(12):1645-1654.
15. Graafland NM, Leijte JA, Valdes Olmos RA, et al. Scanning with 18F-FDG-PET/CT for detection of pelvic nodal involvement in inguinal node-positive penile carcinoma. *Eur Urol*. 2009;56(2):339-345.
16. Leijte JA, Graafland NM, Valdes Olmos RA, et al. Prospective evaluation of hybrid 18F-fluorodeoxyglucose positron emission tomography/computed tomography in staging clinically node-negative patients with penile carcinoma. *BJU Int*. 2009;104(5):640-644.
17. American Joint Committee on Cancer. Penis. In: Amin MB, Edge SB, Greene FL, et al., eds. *AJCC Cancer Staging Manual*. 8th ed. Chicago, IL: Springer; 2017:701-714.
18. Alnajjar HM, Lam W, Bolgeri M, et al. Treatment of carcinoma in situ of the glans penis with topical chemotherapy agents. *Eur Urol*. 2012;62(5):923-928.
19. Lucky M, Murthy KVR, Rogers B, et al. The treatment of penile carcinoma in situ (CIS) within a UK supra-regional network. *BJU Int*. 2015;115(4):595-598.
20. Romero FR, Romero KR, Mattos MA, et al. Sexual function after partial penectomy for penile cancer. *Urology*. 2005;66(6):1292-1295.
21. de Crevoisier R, Slimane K, Sanfilippo N, et al. Long-term results of brachytherapy for carcinoma of the penis confined to the glans (N- or NX). *Int J Radiation Oncol Biol Phys*. 2009;74(4):1150-1156.
22. Ficarra V, Akduman B, Bouchot O, et al. Prognostic factors in penile cancer. *Urology*. 2010;76(2, Suppl):S66-S73.
23. Cabanas RM. An approach for the treatment of penile carcinoma. *Cancer*. 1977;39(2):456-466.

24. Kulkarni JN, Kamat MR. Prophylactic bilateral groin node dissection versus prophylactic radiotherapy and surveillance in patients with N0 and N1-2A carcinoma of the penis. *Eur Urol.* 1994;26(2):123-128.
25. Leijte JAP, Kirrander P, Antonini N, et al. Recurrence patterns of squamous cell carcinoma of the penis: recommendations for follow-up based on a two-centre analysis of 700 patients. *Eur Urol.* 2008;54(1):161-169.
26. Lopes A, Hidalgo GS, Kowalski LP, et al. Prognostic factors in carcinoma of the penis: multivariate analysis of 145 patients treated with amputation and lymphadenectomy. *J Urol.* 1996;156(5):1637-1642.
27. Ornellas AA, Seixas AL, Marota A, et al. Surgical treatment of invasive squamous cell carcinoma of the penis: retrospective analysis of 350 cases. *J Urol.* 1994;151(5):1244-1249.
28. Solsona E, Iborra I, Ricos JV, et al. Corpus cavernosum invasion and tumor grade in the prediction of lymph node condition in penile carcinoma. *Eur Urol.* 1992;22(2):115-118.
29. Theodorescu D, Russo P, Zhang ZF, et al. Outcomes of initial surveillance of invasive squamous cell carcinoma of the penis and negative nodes. *J Urol.* 1996;155(5):1626-1631.
30. Slaton JW, Morgenstern N, Levy DA, et al. Tumor stage, vascular invasion and the percentage of poorly differentiated cancer: independent prognosticators for inguinal lymph node metastasis in penile squamous cancer. *J Urol.* 2001;165(4):1138-1142.
31. Ficarra V, Zattoni F, Artibani W, et al. Nomogram predictive of pathological inguinal lymph node involvement in patients with squamous cell carcinoma of the penis. *J Urol.* 2006;175(5):1700-1704; discussion 4-5.
32. Horenblas S, van Tinteren H. Squamous cell carcinoma of the penis. IV. Prognostic factors of survival: analysis of tumor, nodes and metastasis classification system. *J Urol.* 1994;151(5):1239-1243.
33. Solsona E, Iborra I, Rubio J, et al. Prospective validation of the association of local tumor stage and grade as a predictive factor for occult lymph node micrometastasis in patients with penile carcinoma and clinically negative inguinal lymph nodes. *J Urol.* 2001;165(5):1506-1509.
34. Soria JC, Fizazi K, Piron D, et al. Squamous cell carcinoma of the penis: multivariate analysis of prognostic factors and natural history in monocentric study with a conservative policy. *Ann Oncol.* 1997;8(11):1089-1098.
35. Crawshaw JW, Hadway P, Hoffland D, et al. Sentinel lymph node biopsy using dynamic lymphoscintigraphy combined with ultrasound-guided fine needle aspiration in penile carcinoma. *Br J Radiol.* 2009;82(973):41-48.

36. Hughes B, Leijte J, Shabbir M, et al. Non-invasive and minimally invasive staging of regional lymph nodes in penile cancer. *World J Urol*. 2009;27(2):197-203.
37. Leijte JA, Kroon BK, Valdes Olmos RA, et al. Reliability and safety of current dynamic sentinel node biopsy for penile carcinoma. *Eur Urol*. 2007;52(1):170-177.
38. Grabstald H. Controversies concerning lymph node dissection for cancer of the penis. *Urol Clin North Am*. 1980;7(3):793-799.
39. Horenblas S, van Tinteren H, Delemarre JF, et al. Squamous cell carcinoma of the penis. III. Treatment of regional lymph nodes. *J Urol*. 1993;149(3):492-497.
40. Zargar-Shoshtari K, Djajadiningrat R, Sharma P, et al. Establishing criteria for bilateral pelvic lymph node dissection in the management of penile cancer: lessons learned from an international multicenter collaboration. *J Urol*. 2015;194(3):696-701.

Treatment of Metastatic Penile Cancer: Chemotherapy 34

Abhishek Marballi and Teresa Gray Hayes

Penile cancer is a rare malignancy, representing less than 1% of all cancers in men in the United States. It is relatively more common in parts of Southeast Asia, South America, and Africa. The rate of penile cancer increases with age, the mean age of diagnosis being 60 years. Penile cancer arises from the inner prepuce or glans and squamous cell carcinoma (SCC) accounts for the majority (>95%), although other histological subtypes occur.

Human papillomavirus (HPV) is a risk factor and about 30% to 40% of cases of penile cancer are associated with HPV-related carcinogenesis. HPV 16, HPV 6, and HPV 18 are the most frequent types encountered in penile SCC. There is conflicting data regarding the prognostic implications of presence of HPV. Other risk factors include penile injury, genital warts, presence of phimosis, lack of circumcision, and tobacco exposure.

Penile cancer initially spreads via lymphatics in a very predictable manner. Lymphatic spread from the primary penile tumor can be unilateral or bilateral. The superficial and deep inguinal lymph nodes are the first to be affected, followed by ipsilateral pelvic lymph nodes. Pelvic lymph node spread without ipsilateral inguinal lymph node involvement has never been reported. Involvement of para-aortic and paracaval lymph nodes is considered to be systemic metastatic disease. Distant metastases (e.g., bone, lung, liver, or brain) are rare and detected late in the course of the disease.

The aim of treatment for early stage disease is radical tumor removal with maximal possible organ preservation. Treatment approach depends upon tumor, node, and metastasis (TNM) classification and grade of differentiation.

LOCALLY ADVANCED DISEASE

The 5-year cancer-specific survival is 90% to 100% in patients with pN0 disease, between 70% and 80% in patients with pN1 stage disease, and less than 30% for stage pN2-3 disease (1). In a study by Pandey et al, case records of 128 patients who underwent groin dissection for penile cancer were reviewed (2). It was noted that patients who had metastasis only to inguinal nodes had a 5-year overall survival (OS) of 65%, but patients with pelvic nodal metastasis had a 5-year OS of 0%. On multivariate analysis, the factors adversely influencing survival were: ≥ 4 positive inguinal nodes, bilateral nodal metastases (N2), extranodal extension, and pelvic nodal metastasis (N3). Based on these findings, it is desirable to consider a multimodality approach to patients with these adverse factors. To explore this strategy, a prospective phase 2 trial included 30 patients with N2 or N3 disease without distant metastases. These patients received neoadjuvant paclitaxel 175 mg/m^2 on day 1, ifosfamide 1,200 mg/m^2 days 1 to 3, and cisplatin 25 mg/m^2 on days 1 to 3 (TIP) for four cycles with intent to undergo lymphadenectomy. Results revealed an objective response of 50% with 30% alive at 34 months. There were no chemotherapy-related deaths. OS was significantly associated with response to chemotherapy. Authors recommend neoadjuvant TIP as a part of multimodal treatment in these patients (3). In another prospective clinical trial, patients were treated with bleomycin, methotrexate, and cisplatin. Although an overall response rate of 32% and median OS of 28 weeks were found, the benefits were offset by a 14% treatment-related mortality (4). Since there isn't sufficient data to form conclusions regarding adjuvant chemotherapy, the recommendations are based on extrapolation of neoadjuvant data mentioned earlier. As per National Comprehensive Cancer Network (NCCN) guidelines, adjuvant TIP for four cycles is reasonable for patients who didn't receive preoperative chemotherapy and have any of the high-risk features such as pelvic node metastases, extranodal extension, involvement of bilateral inguinal lymph nodes, or ≥ 4 cm tumor in lymph nodes.

METASTATIC DISEASE

Stage IV penile cancer is defined as N3 (palpable fixed inguinal nodes or involved pelvic lymph nodes) or M1 (distant metastases) according to the TNM system (5). In order to identify prognostic factors, Pond et al conducted a retrospective analysis of 140 patients with locally advanced or metastatic prostate SCC receiving first-line chemotherapy. The multivariate model of poor prognostic factors included visceral metastases and Eastern Cooperative Oncology Group (ECOG) performance status (PS) ≥ 1 for progression-free survival (PFS) and OS. It was noted that patients with one or both risk factors had an OS of 8 and 7 months respectively, whereas for patients with 0 risk factors the median OS was not reached. About 73% of patients received cisplatin-based combination chemotherapy. If all cisplatin-based regimens were combined, there was an improved hazard ratio of 0.49 for survival compared to patients who did not receive cisplatin, after adjusting for visceral metastases and ECOG PS. The conclusion was that ECOG PS ≥ 1 and visceral metastases were poor prognostic factors and cisplatin-based regimens induced better outcomes compared to non–cisplatin-based regimens in patients with advanced penile SCC (6). A retrospective analysis by Di Lorenzo et al included 25 patients with newly diagnosed or recurrent penile cancer not amenable to either radical surgery or neoadjuvant chemotherapy followed by radical intent surgery. All patients received first-line chemotherapy with cisplatin on day 1 followed by 5-fluorouracil (5-FU) as continuous infusion for 4 days every 3 weeks until disease progression or unacceptable toxicity. A median of six cycles were administered and there were no deaths or interruption of treatment for toxicity. Treatment was well tolerated overall. Partial responses were observed in 32% and stable disease in 40% of patients. Median OS was 8 months. The authors concluded that this regimen is associated with a moderate response and tolerated well in patients with metastatic penile SCC (7). Based on extrapolation from neoadjuvant data (3), TIP is the preferred regimen in the metastatic setting with 5-FU + cisplatin as an acceptable alternative.

Endothelial growth factor receptor (EGFR) is highly expressed in penile SCC as demonstrated by a retrospective analysis. Using immunohistochemistry, the expression of EGFR in histological samples of 44 patients with penile SCC was evaluated. Results revealed that 40/44 samples (91%) showed a strong positive expression of EGFR (8). To evaluate efficacy of EGFR-targeted therapy in penile SCC, Carthon et al retrospectively analyzed 24 patients treated at MD Anderson Cancer Center. All patients had penile SCC with clinical T4 or N2, N3 or M1 disease. Of patients, 67% received cetuximab in combination with cytotoxic chemotherapy, mostly a platinum agent. Others received erlotinib or gefitinib. Results revealed a partial response in 23% of patients, with median time to progression (TTP) of 11.3 weeks and median OS of 29.6 weeks. Gefitinib and erlotinib didn't induce objective responses. The most common toxic effect was grade 1 and grade 2 rash. The study concluded that cetuximab has antitumor activity in metastatic penile SCC and may enhance the effect of cisplatin-based chemotherapy (9).

After First-Line Chemotherapy Failure

Out of 30 patients who received neoadjuvant TIP for Tx, N2 or N3, M0 disease as described earlier in the prospective phase 2 trial (3), 19 patients had tumor progression or recurrence. A retrospective analysis evaluated the response to subsequent treatment and survival. Seventeen patients went on to receive salvage therapy. Four patients underwent salvage surgery and all of them experienced disease progression. Only two out of five patients who received bleomycin, methotrexate, and cisplatin had an objective response. There were no other documented responses to systemic therapy. OS was 5.6 months for patients who received cisplatin-based treatment and 4.3 months for those who didn't (10). The conclusion is that patients with recurrent disease or progression after first-line chemotherapy experience poor responses to salvage treatments. With a median survival of less than 6 months, these patients should be placed on clinical trials or referred to hospice.

KEY POINTS

- For locally advanced disease Tx, N2 or N3 without distant metastases: neoadjuvant TIP followed by lymphadenectomy.
- Adjuvant chemotherapy with TIP should be considered for patients with high-risk features such as pelvic node metastases, extranodal extension, involvement of bilateral inguinal lymph nodes, or ≥ 4 cm tumor in lymph nodes.
- For distant metastases or disease not amenable to surgery, palliative TIP is the preferred regimen with 5-FU + cisplatin as an acceptable alternative.
- Penile cancer exhibits high expression of EGFR. Cetuximab has antitumor activity and may enhance effects of platinum-based treatment. Cetuximab may be considered in select patients if not treated previously with a similar class of agent.
- Patients with recurrent disease or progression after first-line chemotherapy respond poorly to salvage treatment and should be placed on clinical trial or referred to hospice.

REFERENCES

1. Bezerra AL, Lopes A, Santiago GH, et al. Human papillomavirus as a prognostic factor in carcinoma of the penis: analysis of 82 patients treated with amputation and bilateral lymphadenectomy. *Cancer.* 2001;91:2315-2321.
2. Pandey D, Mahajan V, Kannan RR. Prognostic factors in node-positive carcinoma of the penis. *J Surg Oncol.* 2006;93:133-138.
3. Pagliaro LC, Williams DL, Daliani D, et al. Neoadjuvant paclitaxel, ifosfamide, and cisplatin chemotherapy for metastatic penile cancer: a phase II study. *J Clin Oncol.* 2010;28(24):3851-3857.
4. Haas GP, Blumenstein BA, Gagliano RG, et al. Cisplatin, methotrexate and bleomycin for the treatment of carcinoma of the penis: a Southwest Oncology Group study. *J Urol.* 1999;161:1823-1825.

5. American Joint Committee on Cancer. Penis. In: Amin MB, Edge SB, Greene FL, et al., eds. *AJCC Cancer Staging Manual,* 8th ed. Chicago, IL: Springer; 2017:701-714.
6. Pond GR, Di Lorenzo G, Necchi A, et al. Prognostic risk stratification derived from individual patient level data for men with advanced penile squamous cell carcinoma receiving first-line systemic therapy. *Urol Oncol.* 2014;32(4):501-508.
7. Di Lorenzo G, Buonerba C, Federico P, et al. Cisplatin and 5-fluorouracil in inoperable, stage IV squamous cell carcinoma of the penis. *BJU Int.* 2012;110(11 Pt B):E661-E666.
8. Börgermann C, Schmitz KJ, Sommer S, et al. Characterization of the EGF receptor status in penile cancer: retrospective analysis of the course of the disease in 45 patients. *Urologe A.* 2009;48(12):1483-1489.
9. Carthon BC, Ng CS, Pettaway CA, Pagliaro LC. Epidermal growth factor receptor-targeted therapy in locally advanced or metastatic squamous cell carcinoma of the penis. *BJU Int.* 2014;113(6):871-877.
10. Wang J, Pettaway CA, Pagliaro LC. Treatment for metastatic penile cancer after first-line chemotherapy failure: analysis of response and survival outcomes. *Urology.* 2015;85(5):1104-1110.

Controversies in the Management of Penile Cancer 35

Guilherme Godoy

INTRODUCTION

Penile cancer is a rare tumor, accounting for only 0.4% to 0.6% of all malignancies in men (1,2). Additionally, it has a profound social-psychological impact, further aggravated by the lack of awareness and public information. Affected men are often embarrassed about their condition, which delays their decision to seek medical attention. The limited number of cases seen by health care providers also contributes to delayed and suboptimal care for these men, especially in areas where supraregional specialized centers do not exist.

Despite all these challenges, basic understanding of the clinical natural history and the management of both primary lesions and regional lymph node metastasis are well defined. The primary tumor starts at the glans, sulcus, or foreskin, and advances to invade deeply into the corpora and urethra, toward the base of the penis. The pattern of metastatic spread is well described and predictable, starting in regional inguinal lymph nodes and progressing, in a stepwise fashion, to pelvic lymph nodes before disseminating to distant sites (3). Some controversies still exist, especially in the management of inguinal and pelvic lymph node metastasis. The following cases illustrate some of these situations.

Case 1: A 53-year-old White Hispanic male was referred to the urologic clinic 1 year after circumcision, with a fungating mass replacing the glans and a 3-cm mobile palpable area of lymphadenopathy in the right inguinal region. He underwent a partial penectomy revealing a pT3 moderately differentiated squamous cell carcinoma (SCC).

Question 1: What should be the laterality and the extent of the inguinal lymph node dissection in patients with unilateral palpable lymphadenopathy?

This case illustrates the rapid progression of the primary tumor. There were inguinal lymph nodes slightly greater than 1 cm in the left side identified by surgical dissection, which were not palpable and nonspecific on imaging staging tests. Intraoperative mapping studies have observed that the lymphatic drainage from penile lesions is bilateral, with considerable crossover between sides (4,5). In this particular case, the left inguinal nodes were negative; however, micrometastases are present in 20% to 25% of nonpalpable nodes. Conversely, palpable inguinal nodes are positive in 50% to 80% of cases (3,6). Therefore, bilateral inguinal lymph node dissection is mandatory for adequate staging and offers potential therapeutic benefit.

Because of concerns with morbidity and complications associated with radical standard inguinal lymph node dissection templates, the use of fine needle aspiration and more limited templates have been proposed. However, in the presence of positive lymph node identified during frozen-section analysis, the procedure should be converted to a standard dissection template. In the abovementioned case, not only was a large lymph node palpable, but the primary tumor had high-risk features (pT3) that would indicate the need for the bilateral inguinal lymph node dissection. In situations like this, in the presence of unilateral palpable disease, limited templates can be performed on the contralateral side with dissection performed only superficially to the *fascia lata*, as long as there is no histological evidence of positive involvement observed during frozen-section analysis (7).

Question 2: He underwent bilateral inguinal lymph node dissection, including the deep inguinal nodes with sartorius muscle transposition flap in the right side and superficial dissection in the left side. A large lymph node (4.5 cm) was positive in the right side, while all lymph nodes from the left side were negative. What is the role of *pelvic* lymph node dissection in the setting of a histologically confirmed positive groin? When is a bilateral pelvic lymphadenectomy indicated?

The role of the pelvic lymph dissection and whether it should be performed bilaterally or ipsilateral to the positive inguinal side are still controversial topics. There is also debate if adjuvant chemotherapy with TIP (paclitaxel, ifosfamide, cisplatin) or chemoradiation following the inguinal or the pelvic lymph node dissection is beneficial. A simplistic approach would be to omit the pelvic lymph node dissection only if the bilateral inguinal lymph node dissection is negative, since skip metastasis has not been reported (8,9). Otherwise, all patients should undergo bilateral pelvic lymph node dissection. Although the presence of positive inguinal lymph nodes suggests the presence of systemic disease, the indication for a pelvic lymph node dissection is based on the potential therapeutic benefit and the lack of effective systemic therapy for advanced disease. Alternatively, a more selective approach would indicate ipsilateral pelvic lymph node dissection only in cases where there is poorly differentiated tumor present in the lymph node, extranodal extension, nodal size greater than 3.5 cm, or more than two lymph nodes involved (10,11). If any of those high-risk features are present in both inguinal regions, a bilateral pelvic lymph node dissection is indicated, each side mandated for ipsilateral pelvic dissection. Recently, a multicenter international study has proposed that, besides the presence of bilateral extranodal extension, the finding of four or more inguinal lymph nodes (both sides combined) would indicate the need for a bilateral pelvic lymph node dissection (12).

Case 2: A 73-year-old African American male had a partial penectomy with negative margins for a pT3 well differentiated SCC. After the resection of the primary tumor, the previously palpable right inguinal lymphadenopathy resolved and became nonpalpable.

Question 3: What is the role of the dynamic sentinel node biopsy (DSNB) in the management of nonpalpable inguinal regions?
In centers where there is appropriate experience and expertise, DSNB can be performed as an alternative to inguinal lymph node dissection in men with clinically nonpalpable nodes, even in the presence of high-risk primary tumors such as the present case (13–15). There has been controversy about

the reproducibility and true utility of the DNSB technique. However, recent refinements of the technique, such as the incorporation of fine needle aspiration under ultrasound guidance, have led to a decrease in the false-negative rate from 19% to 5% (14,16). In centers lacking expertise in the DSNB technique, close surveillance of low-risk primary tumors (Tis, Ta, and T1a), and bilateral inguinal lymph node dissection in the intermediate/high-risk primary tumors (T1b, T2+), are the recommended approaches in men with clinically negative groins.

Question 4: Patient declined the recommendation for a bilateral inguinal lymph node dissection. After 9 months of follow-up, he again developed palpable and mobile lymph nodes in the right inguinal region. Is there a difference between immediate and delayed lymphadenectomy in men with nonpalpable nodes? Is a bilateral lymph node dissection necessary for a late unilateral nodal recurrence?

Evidence suggests that men with clinically negative groins and high-risk primary tumors have better oncological outcomes with immediate bilateral inguinal lymph node dissection than with a delayed dissection after the nodes become palpable. However, when the nodes become palpable during an initial period of observation, an ipsilateral inguinal lymph node dissection may be performed, since absence of disease development in the groin usually suggests freedom from disease on that side. There is debate about the minimum period of observation and also whether this practice should be widely recommended (7,17,18). In the presence of aggressive and bulky unilateral disease (≥4 cm nodes), a contralateral dissection should also be considered (7).

KEY POINTS

- Several areas of debate still exist around the management of penile cancer, mostly related to the management of regional and pelvic lymph nodes.
- A bilateral inguinal lymph node dissection should always be performed in patients with high-risk primary tumors and/or histologically proven palpable nodes.

(continued)

(continued)

- An immediate bilateral inguinal lymph node dissection yields better oncological outcomes than a delayed approach in men with clinically negative groins and high-risk primary tumors.
- When lymphadenopathy develops later in follow-up, unilateral dissection is acceptable, as long as there is an absence of bulky disease (>4 cm lymph nodes).
- The role of the pelvic lymph dissection and whether it should be performed bilaterally or ipsilateral to the positive inguinal side are still controversial topics.
- DSNB is an acceptable approach in men with nonpalpable inguinal nodes, especially with low-risk primary tumors, but only if there is adequate expertise available.

REFERENCES

1. Presti JC. Genital tumors. In: McAninch JW, Lue TF, eds. *Smith and Tanagho's General Urology*. 18th ed. New York, NY: McGraw-Hill/Lange; 2013.
2. Siegel RL, Miller KD, Jemal A. Cancer statistics, 2017. *CA Cancer J Clin*. 2017;67(1):7-30.
3. Pettaway CA, Crook JM, Pagliaro LC. Penile carcinoma. In: Wein AJ, Kavoussi LR, Partin AW, et al., eds. *Campbell-Walsh Urology*. 10th ed. Philadelphia, PA: Elsevier; 2016:846-878.
4. Horenblas S, Jansen L, Meinhardt W, et al. Detection of occult metastasis in squamous cell carcinoma of the penis using a dynamic sentinel node procedure. *J Urol*. 2000;163(1):100-104.
5. Spiess PE, Izawa JI, Bassett R, et al. Preoperative lymphoscintigraphy and dynamic sentinel node biopsy for staging penile cancer: results with pathological correlation. *J Urol*. 2007;177(6):2157-2161.
6. Hegarty PK, Kayes O, Freeman A, et al. A prospective study of 100 cases of penile cancer managed according to European Association of Urology guidelines. *BJU Int*. 2006;98(3):526-531.
7. Hegarty PK, Dinney CP, Pettaway CA. Controversies in ilioinguinal lymphadenectomy. *Urol Clin North Am*. 2010;37(3):421-434.
8. Russo P, Horenblas S. Surgical management of penile carcer. In: Scardino PT, Linehan WM, Zelefsky MJ, et al., eds. *Comprehensive Textbook of Genitourinary Oncology*. 4th ed. Baltimore, MD: Wolters Kluwer–Lippincott Williams & Wilkins; 2011:811-822.

9. Srinivas V, Morse MJ, Herr HW, et al. Penile cancer: relation of extent of nodal metastasis to survival. *J Urol.* 1987;137(5):880-882.
10. Lont AP, Kroon BK, Gallee MPW, et al. Pelvic lymph node dissection for penile carcinoma: extent of Inguinal lymph node involvement as an indicator for pelvic lymph node involvement and survival. *J Urol.* 2007;177(3):947-952.
11. Zhu Y, Zhang SL, Ye DW, et al. Predicting pelvic lymph node metastases in penile cancer patients: a comparison of computed tomography, Cloquet's node, and disease burden of inguinal lymph nodes. *Onkologie.* 2008;31(1-2):37-41.
12. Zargar-Shoshtari K, Djajadiningrat R, Sharma P, et al. Establishing criteria for bilateral pelvic lymph node dissection in the management of penile cancer: lessons learned from an international multicenter collaboration. *J Urol.* 2015;194(3):696-702.
13. Heyns CF, Fleshner N, Sangar V, et al. Management of the lymph nodes in penile cancer. *Urology.* 2010;76(2 suppl 1):S43-S57.
14. Leijte JA, Kroon BK, Valdes Olmos RA, et al. Reliability and safety of current dynamic sentinel node biopsy for penile carcinoma. *Eur Urol.* 2007;52(1):170-177.
15. Ficarra V, Galfano A. Should the dynamic sentinel node biopsy (DSNB) be considered the gold standard in the evaluation of lymph node status in patients with penile carcinoma? *Eur Urol.* 2007;52(1):17-19; discussion 20-21.
16. Kroon BK, Horenblas S, Estourgie SH, et al. How to avoid false-negative dynamic sentinel node procedures in penile carcinoma. *J Urol.* 2004;171(6 Pt 1):2191.
17. Ekstrom T, Edsmyr F. Cancer of the penis: a clinical study of 229 cases. *Acta Chir Scand.* 1958;115(1-2):25-45.
18. Horenblas S. Lymphadenectomy for squamous cell carcinoma of the penis. Part 2: the role and technique of lymph node dissection. *BJU Int.* 2001;88(5):473-483.

Penile Cancer Survivorship Challenges and Issues 36

Spencer Craven and Guilherme Godoy

INTRODUCTION

Cancer of the penis is a rare genitourinary malignancy with a low incidence in Europe and North America (<1 per 100,000), but with a significant presence in South America, Southeast Asia, and Africa, where there is an annual incidence of 2.3 to 8.3 per 100,000 (1). The majority of the malignant penile tumors are classified as squamous cell carcinoma and originate from the inner prepuce, sulcus, or the glans of men in their sixth decade of life. The presence of phimosis and uncircumcised foreskin is strongly associated with penile cancer (odds ratio 11.4) (2). This cancer carries a poor prognosis once it has metastasized and reached advanced stages, but local occurrences can be cured in up to 80% of cases.

Prevention strategies play a unique role in penile cancer management. The majority of the known risk factors are patient dependent and modifiable. For instance, cigarette smoking, presence of uncircumcised foreskin, phimosis, and chronic inflammation have all been identified as common and important risk factors for the development of penile cancer. All of these factors can be modified and controlled with corresponding reduction in the relative risk of associated cancer. The practice of circumcision has been shown to reduce the incidence of penile cancer, but the benefit is only detected when it is performed in the neonatal or prepubertal period, and not during adulthood (2). Indeed, the incidence of penile cancer is lower in regions where the practice is common in neonates. Human papillomavirus (HPV) infection has also been shown to have a clear association with genital warts and genital cancers in both men and women. The advent of the HPV vaccine has led to a substantial decrease in HPV related cancers in women. Although studies have yet to show a similar decrease in men, it can be inferred that increasing HPV vaccination rates among men could greatly reduce the incidence of penile cancer (3). However, in many areas penile cancer is also associated with poor socioeconomic status, and this is perhaps one of the strongest barriers against the implementation of effective prevention strategies.

Treatment for penile cancer has evolved in recent years. With greater concern for preservation of both the urinary and sexual function, and also increasing awareness and attention to the psychological impact of the disease, a series of new techniques have been adopted in the management of these tumors. Especially in the early stages of the disease, less invasive surgical strategies were developed to address both the primary tumor and the regional lymph nodes. The goal was to maintain the oncological adequacy of treatment while reducing the morbidity of the radical surgical resections (4). This is a critical aspect related to the quality of life of penile cancer survivors, and is greatly impacted by the type of treatment that they receive. In patients undergoing minimally invasive procedures such as laser ablation or glansectomy, sexual function is maintained in a good proportion of the penile cancer survivors, reported to be 100% and 79%, respectively. After partial penectomy, although over 50% of patients still reported enough erectile function to allow sexual intercourse, there was a marked reduction in sexual satisfaction (2). In total penectomy patients, phallic reconstruction is the only option for regaining sexual function. Whichever treatment is chosen, practitioners should pay special attention to their patients' psychosocial needs during the management of this disease. Most treatment providers don't spend much time discussing sexual function and assessing feelings of shame or inadequacy after treatment, but these issues must be addressed for patients to regain their quality of life. As part of a multidisciplinary team approach, psychological assessment before treatment and during the continued follow-up period is a critical component in this population.

Recurrence rates depend on the disease stage at presentation and the chosen method of treatment. Local recurrence is highest when associated with organ-preserving treatment strategies, with a rate of up to 27% in the first 2 years. Therefore, it is imperative that these patients have a close surveillance follow-up during the first 2 to 3 years after treatment. For patients undergoing partial penectomy, the risk of local recurrence is much lower, at 4% to 5%. Nodal recurrence rates are very low in patients with negative nodes after invasive staging (2.3%), while in those with positive nodes without adjuvant treatment the risk is as high as 19% (2). Recurrence in the inguinal region represents very poor prognosis, with median survival less than 6 months. Pelvic lymph node metastasis is an ominous finding, with a 5-year survival of 10% (5,6). Overall, most recurrences will occur within the first 2 years (74%) and almost all within the first 5 years of follow-up after treatment (92.2%). For this reason, the European Association of Urology recommends that all patients undergo follow-up for at least 5 years, with a more intensive period in the first 2 years.

An adequate follow-up schedule is dictated by the initial stage of the primary tumor, the status of regional lymph nodes, and the initial treatment modality received. In all patients it should include a clinical exam of the penis and the bilateral inguinal regions. Routine imaging may not be indicated in patients with early stage of disease and negative groins, but it may help in obese patients where physical examination is limited, or upon positive clinical findings. For patients with N2 or N3 disease, routine imaging of chest, abdomen, and pelvis is recommended at regular intervals (3–6 months) in the first 2 years of follow-up and at the discretion of the treating physician thereafter (2).

KEY POINTS

- Prevention strategies in penile cancer are an important consideration and can include interventions such as HPV vaccination, circumcision, and smoking cessation.
- Organ-preserving treatments provide better quality of life outcomes and should always be considered.
- All penile cancer survivors should have psychosocial assessment and support during diagnosis, treatment, and follow-up.
- Local recurrence rates are important in this disease, and all patients should have a close follow-up for at least 2 to 5 years.

REFERENCES

1. Barnholtz-Sloan JS, Maldonado JL, Pow-sang J, et al. Incidence trends in primary malignant penile cancer. *Urol Oncol.* 2007;25:361-367.
2. Hakenberg OW, Comperat EM, Minhas S, et al. EAU guidelines on penile cancer: 2014 update. *Eur Urol.* 2015;67:142-150.
3. Diorio GJ, Giuliano AR. The role of human papilloma virus in penile carcinogenesis and preneoplastic lesions: a potential target for vaccination and treatment strategies. *Urol Clin N Am.* 2016;43:419-425.
4. Burnett AL. Penile preserving and reconstructive surgery in the management of penile cancer. *Nat Rev.* 2016;13:249-257.
5. Heyns DF, Fleshner N, Sangar V, et al. Management of the lymph nodes in penile cancer. *Urology.* 2010;76:43-57.
6. Baumgarten AS, Alhammali E, Hakky TS, et al. Salvage surgical resection for isolated locally recurrent inguinal lymph node metastasis of penile cancer: international study collaboration. *J Urol.* 2014;192:760-764.

Index

abiraterone, 51
ablation, 74, 91–92, 257
ACS. *See* American Cancer Society
ACTH. *See* adrenocorticotropic hormone
active surveillance (AS), 39, 219
 for prostate cancer patients, 10–14
 of small renal tumors, 93
adjunct therapy
 for androgen deprivation therapy-related bone demineralization, 65–66
 for bone metastases, 66–67
adjuvant chemotherapy, 227
 for bladder cancers, 189
adrenocorticotropic hormone (ACTH), 59
ADT. *See* androgen deprivation therapy
AFP. *See* alpha-fetoprotein
AJCC. *See* American Joint Committee on Cancer
alpha-fetoprotein (AFP), 215
alpha particle emitters, 55
American Cancer Society (ACS), 7, 44
American Joint Committee on Cancer (AJCC), 9, 16, 128, 225
 bladder cancer staging, 159, 177
 penile cancer staging, 255–256
 prostate cancer staging, 11
American Society for Radiation Oncology (ASTRO), 22, 40
American Society of Clinical Oncology (ASCO), 30, 44, 219
American Urological Association (AUA), 7, 21, 27, 119, 210
 guidelines for prostate cancer, 10
 risk stratification, 161–162
analgesics, 74
androgen deprivation therapy (ADT), 23, 43, 47, 59, 69, 70, 71
 chemohormonal therapy, 49
 intermittent versus continuous, 29–30, 60–62
 medical castration, 48
 metabolic and cardiovascular effects of, 73
 related bone demineralization, adjunct therapy for, 65–66
 surgical orchiectomy, 48
androgen synthesis inhibitors, 51–52
antiandrogen withdrawal, 51
AS. *See* active surveillance
ASCO. *See* American Society of Clinical Oncology
ASTRO. *See* American Society for Radiation Oncology
atezolizumab, 143, 199
AUA. *See* American Urological Association
Australasian Germ Cell Trial Group, 245
axitinib, 99, 119

284 INDEX

Bacillus Calmette-Guérin (BCG), 137
  for bladder cancer, 170, 206
  intolerance of, 171–172
  refractory disease, 172
Balkan nephropathy, 123
BCG. *See* Bacillus Calmette-Guérin
BCR. *See* biochemical relapse
BEP. *See* bleomycin, etoposide, and cisplatin
beta particle emitters, 55
BHD. *See* Birt–Hogg–Dubé syndrome
bicalutamide, 51
bilateral inguinal lymph node dissection, 275, 276
biochemical relapse (BCR), 23–25
  definition of, 27
  incidence of, 28
  radiation therapy, 21–22
  radical prostatectomy, 21
  treatment of, 28
Birt–Hogg–Dubé syndrome (BHD), 84
bisphosphonates, 67
bladder cancer
  adjuvant chemotherapy, 189
  American Urological Association risk stratification, 161–162
  Bacillus Calmette-Guérin for, 170, 171, 206
  bladder preservation, 189–190
  carboplatin-based chemotherapy, 182–183
  CT urogram, 164, 166
  cystectomy, 172–173
  cystoscopy, 164, 165
  enhanced recovery after surgery, 184
  gemcitabine, 170
  immune checkpoint inhibitors, 199–201
  intraoperative frozen section, 185
  management, controversies in, 203–206
  mitomycin C, 169
  muscle invasive, 210–211
  narrow band imaging, 166, 168
  neoadjuvant chemotherapy, 180–182
  nonmuscle invasive, 209–210
  non-urothelial cancers, 158
  pelvic lymphadenectomy, 206
  photodynamic diagnosis, 166
  progression risk, 178
  radiation therapy, 190–191
  radical cystectomy, 183, 203–205
  risk factors, 162–163
  second-line chemotherapy, 197–199
  signs and symptoms, 163
  surveillance, importance of, 191
  TNM staging system, 158–161, 179–180
  transurethral resection of bladder tumor, 168, 169
  2004 WHO grading system, 158
  urinary diversion, 185–188
  urine cytology, 163–164
  urothelial carcinoma, 157, 158
  valrubicin, 170
bladder preservation, 189–190
bleomycin, 238, 245, 268
bleomycin, etoposide, and cisplatin (BEP), 220, 221, 245
bone demineralization, ADT-related, 65–66
bone metastases
  adjunct therapy for, 66–67
  pain from, 74
bone-targeted radiopharmaceuticals, 55
brachytherapy, 15, 16, 23, 258, 259

cabazitaxel, 54
CADT. *See* continuous androgen deprivation therapy
Cancer of the Prostate Strategic Urologic Research Endeavor (CaPSURE), 70
cancer recurrence, 119–120
CaPSURE. *See* Cancer of the Prostate Strategic Urologic Research Endeavor
carboplatin-based chemotherapy, 182–183

INDEX

castration resistant disease
  androgen synthesis inhibitors, 51–52
  antiandrogen withdrawal, 51
  bone-targeted radiopharmaceuticals, 55
  chemotherapy, 53–54
  enzalutamide, 52–53
  first-generation antiandrogens, 51
  immunotherapy— sipuleucel-T, 53
castration sensitive disease, 47–49
cetuximab, 270
chemohormonal therapy, 49
chemotherapy, 221, 275
  for castration resistant prostate cancer, 53–54
  first-line chemotherapy options, 141–143
  second-line chemotherapy options, 197–199, 246–247
chromophobe carcinoma, 80
chronic kidney disease (CKD), 91
cigarette smoking, penile cancer and, 254
cisplatin, 268, 269, 270
cisplatin-based combination chemotherapy, 197, 220, 245, 269
CKD. See chronic kidney disease
clear cell carcinoma, 80
CN. See cytoreductive nephrectomy
collecting duct tumors, 80–81
conditional survival, 154
continent cutaneous diversion, 187
continuous androgen deprivation therapy (CADT), 60–62
corticosteroids, 74
Cowden disease, 85
creatinine clearance, first-line chemotherapy options with, 143
cryoablation, 92, 113
cryotherapy, 17, 23, 91
cryptorchidism, 235
CT urogram, 125, 135, 138, 164, 166

cystectomy, 172, 183, 203, 210, 211
cystoscopy, 127, 154, 164, 165, 166
cytokines, 236
cytoreductive nephrectomy (CN), 104–105
cytotoxic chemotherapy, 236

ddMVAC. See dose-dense Methotrexate + Vinblastine + Doxorubicin + Cisplatin
degarelix, 48
delayed intervention and surveillance for small renal masses (DISSRM), 93
denosumab, 66, 67
DHT. See dihydrotestosterone
digital rectal examination (DRE), 5, 9, 38
dihydrotestosterone (DHT), 59
DISSRM. See delayed intervention and surveillance for small renal masses
docetaxel, 49, 53, 54
dose-dense methotrexate + vinblastine + doxorubicin + cisplatin (ddMVAC), 141, 142
DRE. See digital rectal examination
DSNB. See dynamic sentinel node biopsy
dynamic sentinel node biopsy (DSNB), 260, 261, 275–276

early stage prostate cancer, 9
  active surveillance, 10–14
  biochemical relapse of, 21–25, 27–30
  focal ablation, 17
  localized prostate cancer, 39
  management, controversies in, 37–40
  multimodal use of radiation, 17
  prostate cancer screening, 37–39
  proton therapy, 40
  radiation therapy, 15–17
  radical prostatectomy, 14–15
  survivorship challenges, 43–44

early stage prostate cancer (*cont.*)
  therapy complications, 33–35
  treatment modalities for, 18
Eastern Cooperative Oncology
    Group (ECOG), 269
EAU. *See* European Association of
    Urology
EBRT. *See* external beam
    radiation therapy
ECOG. *See* Eastern Cooperative
    Oncology Group
EGFR. *See* endothelial growth
    factor receptor
endothelial growth factor
    receptor (EGFR), 270
enhanced recovery after surgery
    (ERAS), 184
enzalutamide, 52, 53
EORTC. *See* European
    Organization for Research
    and Treatment of Cancer
ERAS. *See* enhanced recovery
    after surgery
erectile dysfunction, 34–35, 75
erlotinib, 270
ERSPC trial. *See* European
    Randomized Study of
    Screening for Prostate Cancer
etoposide, 239, 246
European Association of Urology
    (EAU), 154
European Organization for
    Research and Treatment
    of Cancer (EORTC)
    30881, 103
European Randomized Study
    of Screening for Prostate
    Cancer (ERSPC) trial, 5, 6, 38
external beam radiation therapy
    (EBRT), 15, 16, 23, 27, 28,
    258, 259

fatigue, 73–74
fertility, testicular cancer on,
    236–237
first-generation antiandrogens,
    70–71
first-line chemotherapy options
    for advanced urothelial
    carcinoma, 142
  with creatinine clearance, 143
  dose-dense methotrexate +
    vinblastine + doxorubicin +
    cisplatin, 141, 142
  gemcitabine plus cisplatin, 141
  in HER2-positive cancer,
    142–143
FLCN. *See* folliculin gene
fluorouracil, 269
flutamide, 51
focal ablation, 17
folliculin gene (FLCN), 84

GC. *See* gemcitabine plus
    cisplatin
GC plus bevacizumab, in
    metastatic urothelial
    cancer, 144
GCTs. *See* germ cell tumors
gefitinib, 270
gemcitabine, 170
gemcitabine plus cisplatin
    (GC), 141
  plus bevacizumab, in metastatic
    urothelial cancer, 144
Genito-Urinary Group of the
    French Federation of Cancer
    Centers (GETUG), 245
germ cell tumors (GCTs), 215,
    221, 225, 243–244
GETUG. *See* Genito-Urinary
    Group of the French
    Federation of Cancer
    Centers
GFR. *See* glomerular
    filtration rate
Gleason score, 9, 10, 12, 22, 23
glomerular filtration rate (GFR),
    117, 125
gonadotropin releasing hormone
    (GnRH) agonists, 48

HDCT. *See* high-dose
    chemotherapy
hereditary leiomyomatosis
    and renal cell carcinoma
    (HLRCC), 84
hereditary papillary renal cell
    carcinoma (HPRCC), 83–84

HER2-positive cancer, first-line chemotherapy options in, 142–143
HIFU. *See* high-intensity focused ultrasound
high-dose bolus IL-2, 98
high-dose chemotherapy (HDCT), 246
high-intensity focused ultrasound (HIFU), 17, 113–114
HIV and HPV infection, penile cancer, 254
HLRCC. *See* hereditary leiomyomatosis and renal cell carcinoma
hormonal therapy, 100
HPRCC. *See* hereditary papillary renal cell carcinoma
HPV. *See* human papillomavirus
human papillomavirus (HPV), 267, 279–280
hydrocortisone, 52
hypospadias, 235
hypoxia inducible factor (HIF-1α), 130

IAD. *See* intermittent androgen deprivation
IADT. *See* intermittent androgen deprivation therapy
ICG. *See* indocyanine green
ICIs. *See* immune checkpoint inhibitors
IFNa. *See* interferon alpha
ifosfamide, 268
ileal conduit diversion, 187
immune checkpoint inhibitors (ICIs), 199–201
immunotherapy, 53, 98–99, 170–171
impotence, 35
IMRT. *See* intensity modulated radiation therapy
indocyanine green (ICG), 114
infertility, 235, 236
inguinal lymph node, 255, 259–262, 267–268, 274–276
intensity modulated radiation therapy (IMRT), 16

interferon alpha (IFN-α), 98
intermittent androgen ablation, in metastatic prostate cancer, 59–62
intermittent androgen deprivation (IAD), 30
intermittent androgen deprivation therapy (IADT), 60–62
International Collaboration of Trialists Study, 181
International Prostate Symptom Score (IPSS), 212
IPSS. *See* International Prostate Symptom Score

ketoconazole, 52
kidney cancer, 117–120
  Birt–Hogg–Dubé syndrome, 84
  chromophobe carcinomas, 80
  clear cell carcinoma, 80
  collecting duct tumors, 80–81
  Cowden disease, 85
  genetic and familial predisposition and, 81
  oncocytomas, 80
  papillary carcinoma, 80
  polycystic kidney disease, 85
  renal cell carcinoma. *See* renal cell carcinoma
  tuberous sclerosis complex, 85
  tumors of kidney, 81
  von Hippel–Lindau syndrome, 82–83

LND. *See* lymph node dissection
localized prostate cancer, treatment of, 39
long-term effects, of targeted agents, 118–119
LVI. *See* lymphovascular invasion
lymphadenectomy, 151, 206, 268, 274
lymphadenopathy, 262, 273–274
lymph node dissection (LND), 103, 137
lymphovascular invasion (LVI), 129

MDRD. *See* modification of diet in renal disease
medical castration, 48, 60
metabolic syndrome, 237
metastatic prostate cancer
  androgen deprivation therapy for, 47
  castration resistant disease, 51–55
  castration sensitive disease, 47–49
  intermittent androgen ablation in, 59–62
  management, controversies in, 69–71
  survivorship challenges and issues, 73–75
  treatment options for, 50
metastatic renal cell carcinoma (mRCC), 104
methotrexate, 268
methotrexate, vinblastine, adriamycin, cisplatin (MVAC), 181, 182, 199
MIBC. *See* muscle-invasive bladder cancer
mitomycin C (MMC), 169
MMC. *See* mitomycin C
modification of diet in renal disease (MDRD), 118
Mohs micrographic surgery, 257–258
mRCC. *See* metastatic renal cell carcinoma
mTOR inhibitors, 99–100
muscle-invasive bladder cancer (MIBC), 158–161, 179, 210–211
MVAC. *See* methotrexate, vinblastine, adriamycin, cisplatin

narrow band imaging (NBI), 166, 168
National Comprehensive Cancer Network (NCCN), 10, 12, 143, 154
NBI. *See* narrow band imaging

NCCN. *See* National Comprehensive Cancer Network
NCCN Clinical Practice Guidelines in Oncology (NCCN Guidelines®), 199, 203, 205, 206
near-infrared fluorescence (NIRF), 114–115
neoadjuvant chemotherapy, 150, 180–182
nephron-sparing surgery (NSS), 106–107, 114
  adjuvant therapy, 137–138
  low-risk and high-risk tumors, 136
  lymph node dissections, 137
  radical nephroureterectomy, 136–137
  treatment, 138
nerve blocks, 74
neuropathic pain agents, 74
nilutamide, 51
NIRF. *See* near-infrared fluorescence
NMIBC. *See* nonmuscle-invasive bladder cancer
nodal involvement, location of, 104
non-clear cell carcinoma, systemic therapy of, 100
nonmuscle-invasive bladder cancer (NMIBC), 158–161, 209–210
  American Urological Association risk stratification, 161–162
  radical cystectomy for, 172
  signs and symptoms, 163
  transurethral resection of bladder tumor, 168
nonregional lymph node, 221
nonseminomatous germ cell tumors (NSGCTs)
  early-stage disease, 225–228
  good-risk, 228–229
  intermediate-risk, 229
  poor-risk, 229

relapsed/refractory disease, 229–231
surveillance, 231–232
NSGCTs. *See* nonseminomatous germ cell tumors
NSS. *See* nephron-sparing surgery

oncocytoma, 80
orthotopic neobladders, 188
osteoclast inhibition, 65, 66
osteoporosis, ADT-related, 66
ototoxicity, 238

paclitaxel, 197, 268
palliative chemotherapy, 222, 231
papillary carcinoma, 80
papillary urothelial neoplasm of low malignant potential (PUNLMP), 158
partial nephrectomy (PN), 90–91
pazopanib, 98, 99, 118–119
PCKD. *See* polycystic kidney disease
PCOS. *See* Prostate Cancer Outcomes Study
PDD. *See* photodynamic diagnosis
PeIN. *See* penile intraepithelial neoplasia
pelvic lymphadenectomy, 206, 274
pelvic lymph node dissection, 183, 261, 267, 274–275
penile cancer, 267
  ablation techniques, 257
  after first-line chemotherapy failure, 270
  biopsy, 255
  brachytherapy, 258–259
  cigarette smoking, 254
  circumcision, 257
  external beam radiation therapy, 258–259
  histopathologic subtypes of, 251, 252, 254
  HIV and HPV infection, 254
  locally advanced disease, 268
  lymphatics, 267
  management, controversies in, 273–276
  metastatic disease, 269–270
  Mohs micrographic surgery, 257–258
  phimosis and uncircumcised foreskin, 253
  premalignant lesions, 252, 253
  prevention strategies in, 279
  recurrence rates, 280–281
  regional lymph nodes, management of, 259–262
  surgical resection, 258
  TNM staging, 255–256
  treatment for, 257, 280
  tumors classification, 279
penile intraepithelial neoplasia (PeIN), 254
percutaneous vertebral augmentation, 74
PFS. *See* progression-free survival
phimosis, 253
photodynamic diagnosis (PDD), 166–167
PLCO screening trial. *See* Prostate, Lung, Colorectal and Ovarian Cancer (PLCO) screening trial
PN. *See* partial nephrectomy
polycystic kidney disease (PCKD), 85
progestins, 75
progression-free survival (PFS), 269
Prostate Cancer Outcomes Study (PCOS), 33
prostate cancer screening, 3, 37–39
  impact of, 5–6
  risks associated with, 6–7
Prostate, Lung, Colorectal and Ovarian Cancer (PLCO) screening trial, 5, 6, 38
prostate-specific antigen (PSA), 9, 21–23, 27, 30, 69–70
  digital rectal examination, 5
  efficacy of, 5
  impact of, 5–6
  management of, 22
  risks associated with, 6–7
  screening, 3–7

prostate-specific antigen (PSA) (cont.)
  testing in malignancy, 4–5
  variations of, 4
prostatic urethral disease, 211
proton therapy, 40
PSA. *See* prostate-specific antigen
PSA doubling time (PSADT), 28, 29
PSADT. *See* PSA doubling time
psoralen plus ultraviolet A radiation, 254
PTEN hamartoma tumor syndrome, 85
PUNLMP. *See* papillary urothelial neoplasm of low malignant potential

QOL. *See* quality of life
quality of life (QOL), 29, 30, 60, 61

radiation exposure, 239
radiation therapy (RT), 23, 74, 101, 220, 258–259
  biochemical relapse after, 21–22
  for bladder cancers, 190
  for prostate cancer, 15–17
radical cystectomy, for bladder cancers, 172, 183, 203–205
radical inguinal orchiectomy, 219, 225
radical nephroureterectomy (RNU), 136–138, 151, 153
radical prostatectomy (RP), 14–15, 21, 27
radiofrequency ablation (RFA), for renal cell carcinoma, 91–92
radiopharmaceuticals, bone-targeted, 55
radium-223, 55
RCC. *See* renal cell carcinoma
regional lymph nodes, and penile cancer, 259–262
renal cell carcinoma (RCC), 113, 147
  ablative techniques, 91–92
  active surveillance, 93
  chemotherapy and hormonal therapy, 100
  classification of, 79
  immunotherapy, 98
  initial assessment of small renal mass, 89–90
  partial nephrectomy, 90–91
  renal mass biopsy, 93–94
  surgical management of, 103–110
  systemic therapy of non-clear cell carcinoma, 100
renal dysfunction, 238
  long-term surveillance for, 118
  nephrectomy, 117–118
renal insufficiency, carboplatin-based chemotherapy, 182–183
renal mass biopsy, 93–94
retroperitoneal lymph node dissection (RPLND), 221, 226, 243–245
RFA. *See* radiofrequency ablation
RNU. *See* radical nephroureterectomy
robotic-assisted laparoscopic prostatectomy, 14
RP. *See* radical prostatectomy
RPLND. *See* retroperitoneal lymph node dissection
RT. *See* radiation therapy

salvage therapy, 28
  after radical prostatectomy, 23
  definitive radiation therapy, 23–25
sarcomatoid renal cell carcinoma, 81
SCC. *See* squamous cell carcinoma
SDH gene. *See* succinate dehydrogenase gene
secondary malignancy, risk of, 239
second-line chemotherapy, 197–199, 246–247
semen cryopreservation, 237
seminoma
  early stage, 219–220
  germ cell tumors, 215
  late stage, 221–222
  serum tumor markers, 216–218
  stage II, 220–221
  stage III, 221–222

serum tumor markers (STMs), 216–218
sipuleucel-T, 53
small cell cancer of prostate, 55–56
small renal mass (SRM), initial assessment of, 89–90
sMVAC. *See* standard MVAC
sorafenib, 118
squamous cell carcinoma (SCC), 158, 251, 267, 270, 279
SRM. *See* small renal mass
standard MVAC (sMVAC), 141
STMs. *See* serum tumor markers
stress incontinence, 34
stress urinary incontinence (SUI), 33, 34
succinate dehydrogenase (SDH) gene, 85–86
SUI. *See* stress urinary incontinence
sunitinib, 118
surgical bilateral orchiectomy, 60
surgical orchiectomy, 48
survivorship, 211–212
systemic therapy of non-clear cell carcinoma, 100

TCC. *See* urothelial carcinoma
TCGA. *See* The Cancer Genome Atlas
testicular cancer, 215, 235
  cardiovascular, 237–238
  fertility effects of, 236
  pulmonary, 238
  renal dysfunction, 238
  reproductive challenges in, 235
  serum tumor markers in, 216–218
  stages of, 217
testosterone, 48, 51, 59–60
The Cancer Genome Atlas (TCGA), 178
therapy complications, treatment of
  erectile dysfunction, 34–35
  urinary incontinence, 33–34
TIGER trial, 230

TNM staging system, 9
  for bladder cancers, 158–161, 179–180
  penile cancer, 255–256
transitional cell carcinoma (TCC). *See* urothelial carcinoma
transurethral resection (TUR), 190
transurethral resection of bladder tumor (TURBT), 168, 169
TSC. *See* tuberous sclerosis complex
tuberous sclerosis complex (TSC), 85
tumor marker elevation, 228
tumors of kidney, 81
TUR. *See* transurethral resection
TURBT. *See* transurethral resection of bladder tumor
2004 WHO grading system, bladder neoplasms, 158

uncircumcised foreskin, 253
United States Preventive Services Task Force (USPSTF), 7
upper tract urothelial cancer (UTUC), 123
  CT urogram, 125
  cystoscopy, 127
  cytology and tumor markers, 126
  epidemiology, 123
  etiology, 123–124
  GC plus bevacizumab, 144
  imaging, 125–126
  lymphadenectomy, 151
  metastatectomy in, 147, 148, 150
  neoadjuvant therapy, 150
  nephron-sparing surgical approaches. *See* nephron-sparing surgery
  pathology, 128
  physical and laboratory examination, 125
  prognosis, 129–130
  radical nephroureterectomy, 151
  risk stratification, 135
  signs and symptoms, 124
  staging, 128
  survival rates, 153
  ureteroscopy, 127

urinary diversion, 185–188
urinary incontinence, 33–34
urine cytology, 163–164
urothelial carcinoma (UC), 153. *See also* upper tract urothelial cancer
USPSTF. *See* United States Preventive Services Task Force
UTUC. *See* upper tract urothelial cancer

valrubicin, 170, 171
vascular endothelial growth factor (VEGF), 83, 98–99
vasomotor symptoms, 74–75
VEGF. *See* vascular endothelial growth factor
VeIP. *See* vinblastine/ifosfamide/cisplatin
venous thromboembolic events (VTE), 184
VHL syndrome. *See* von Hippel–Lindau syndrome
vinblastine/ifosfamide/cisplatin (VeIP), 229, 231, 246
von Hippel–Lindau (VHL) syndrome, 80, 82–83, 91
VTE. *See* venous thromboembolic events

zoledronic acid, 67

Made in the USA
Monee, IL
03 May 2026

49437774R00174